FIERCE

joy

Cover & Layout Design: Elina Diaz

For permission requests, please contact the publisher at:
Mango Publishing Group
2850 Douglas Road, 2nd Floor
Coral Gables, FL 33134 USA
info@mango.bz

For special orders, quantity sales, course adoptions and corporate sales, please email the publisher at sales@mango.bz. For trade and wholesale sales, please contact Ingram Publisher Services at customer.service@ingramcontent.com or +1.800.509.4887.

Fierce Joy: Choosing Brave over Perfect to Find My True Voice

Library of Congress Cataloging
ISBN: (print) 978-1-63353-988-4 (ebook) 978-1-63353-989-1
Library of Congress Control Number: 2019935680
BISAC category code: SEL021000 SELF-HELP / Motivational & Inspirational

Printed in the United States of America

FIERCE

joy

Choosing Brave over Perfect to Find My True Voice

SUSIE CALDWELL RINEHART

mango
PUBLISHING
CORAL GABLES

PRAISE FOR *FIERCE JOY*

"Breathtaking. Raw. Real. This memoir is about what it means to have a voice. When Susie loses her ability to speak, she learns to listen to herself. Honest and poignant, this book also had me laughing out loud."

—Jen Pastiloff, author of *On Being Human* and founder of *The Manifest-Station*

"This stunning memoir wakes us up to the kind of happiness that is possible when we are brave enough to go after it. At the heart of this big, brilliant story is this: You are already enough. This book is wise and revolutionary. It changed my life."

—Christine Carter, author of *Raising Happiness* and *The Sweet Spot*

"Powerful, honest, riveting. What happens when a crisis forces you to give up perfectionism and self-worth through doing? Susie Rinehart's story of survival is a gift to any woman who longs to free herself of the shackles of 'not-enough.' "

—Rachel Simmons, author of *Enough As She Is*

"After reading an excerpt from this book, I was immediately gripped. This is a powerful book for anyone who struggles with perfectionism. The authors reminds us that leading a courageous life means moving forward...even when you don't feel 'perfect' or 'completely ready' yet."

—Alexandra Franzen, author of *You Are Going to Survive* and *So This Is the End*

"This is a powerful story about a woman daring to fight for a life that is big, buoyant, and brilliant. She shows us that we can live lightly in dark times, if we dare to make space for joy."

—Becca Anderson, author of *The Book of Awesome Women* and *Prayers for Hard Times*

"A fundamental shift in the spiritual journey occurs when we realize the inherent gift that lies in speaking from the heart. In *Fierce Joy: Choosing Brave over Perfect to Find My True Voice*, Susie Caldwell Rinehart beautifully captures the spiritual freedom in coming to know what she once viewed as vulnerable is actually the most powerful: when we speak from the heart, we are rooted in truth—our own truth—when what we say, what we do and what we believe are in complete harmony. Susie's story shows us how to transform pain into heart-centered instructions for living our best life."

—Bridgitte Jackson-Buckley, author of *The Gift of Crisis*

"Extraordinary memoir full of hard-won wisdom. This book is about what it means to be human, and what lies beneath our fears if we dare to look."

—Brad Wetzler, former editor, *Outside* magazine, writing coach

"Uplifting and loaded with practical wisdom on how to come out of a crisis with more, not less."

—Suleika Jaouad, *New York Times* "Life, Interrupted" columnist

This book is dedicated to my parents,
C. Douglas Caldwell & Marilyn French Caldwell
for love, and for encouraging me to put safety third.

Table of Contents

PRELUDE

August 18, 2016

I lie here after thirty-six hours of brain surgery wondering, *Who am I?* I am not a wife, not a mother, not a leader, not an athlete. I am a lump in a bed. I can't even help my daughter make breakfast.

I have always identified with the hero role. When I go to the movies, I don't just watch Indiana Jones, I *am* Indiana Jones. I am Jason Bourne. I am Katniss Everdeen. I am never the one standing by, wringing her hands, waiting for the hero to come. I am out there, in the adventure, making things happen. I have plenty of courage. I get shit done. I start companies and lead schools. I win races. I can push through anything. I am not even sure I am alive unless I am striving to make something happen. But there are consequences to pushing, striving, fixing, saving everything and everyone. Right now, my health is at risk. If I don't find a different way, I'll die.

Before now, I never thought I was a perfectionist. My house is too messy. Perfectionists don't go to the grocery store without makeup, in their giraffe pajamas. But when it comes to the stuff that matters— relationships and work—I see now that I am a perfectionist. I never believe I am good enough. I judge myself and I judge others. I get stuck looking for the single, right way beyond criticism to success, before even beginning. I loop around the same questions: *Am I in the right job? Do we live in the right place? Are the kids in the right schools?* I assume that if I do things "right," my family will be safe. No one will get hurt. I act as if life is a Sunday crossword puzzle and I have the only pencil. I put so much pressure on myself that I get sick.

This time, my health isn't just telling me to slow down. It's telling me to transform completely.

The trick is my journey feels like the opposite of a hero's journey. While the classic hero is called to adventure, I am called to lie down and let go. But like the hero, I resist. Lying down doesn't feel brave. It makes me feel useless. I grew up wanting to make everyone proud of me. *How, if not by doing and achieving, do I earn my spot on this beautiful earth? How does anyone?*

My husband Kurt comes to check on me. I am propped up in bed in a head bandage to prevent spinal fluid leakage, and a neck brace to protect my skull-to-shoulder fusion from breaking. I am supposed to be sleeping. Instead I am on my phone, searching the internet for a way out of my current situation.

"What are you looking for?" Kurt asks.

"Lindsey Vonn's workout schedule, after her knee surgery," I say.

Kurt laughs and asks, "You're just days out of surgery and you want to work out like an Olympic downhill skier?"

"I am tired of sitting here, doing nothing. Strong people get up and do something to heal faster. They don't just lie here and wait."

"Is that true? I bet if Lindsey Vonn had two craniotomies and a neck fusion, she'd lie down for a few days."

I am not convinced. The only way I know to get through something difficult is to get back up and push through the pain. I feel like if I just work harder, I can throw off the bed covers, rip off the neck brace, and go home.

In the hero's journey, the hero has sword fights and lightsaber battles to fend off bad guys. My battles are internal. I fend off fear and anxiety. I barely move an inch.

Do I deserve to be here if I can't do anything?

Let's look back in order to go forward.
It helps to start at the beginning.

PART I

NEVER ENOUGH

1

I come from a long line of strong women. My mother's mother taught me to hold a shovel; my father's mother taught me to hold a cigarette. My mother taught me to hold my own. Her motto was, "Love many. Trust few. Always paddle your own canoe." They were widowers and divorcées, single mothers who worshipped hard work and self-reliance. They loved me deeply, fiercely. In their eyes, there was nothing I could not do.

These brave women raised me to believe that I could be anything I wanted to be. But the way I internalized that message was that I must be great at everything. And there were many times that I didn't feel capable of being great. All I ever saw were the outer, perfect performances of women in my life: my grandmother, receiving awards for her athleticism; my mother, in a black graduation gown, receiving her second advanced degree; my stepmother, smiling brightly as she effortlessly prepared a five-course meal. I never heard about their struggles, so I thought that the confusion I experienced was uniquely mine. I assumed everyone else knew exactly what she was doing.

My daughter, at ten, believes that she must be great at everything, too. She and I understand that women are praised for their beauty or their extraordinary accomplishments. When we don't feel beautiful and when we aren't the top performer, we don't question our culture's values—we question our worth. One evening, she sat in the fetal position on our couch, refusing to go to dance class.

"I'm not good enough. I'll never be good enough," she said.

"Ouch," I responded, and tried to get eye contact, but she was looking down and away. I knew that she didn't get the part she desperately wanted in the winter show. But to her, it wasn't just a setback. It was proof that she was flawed, even broken. She felt that if she didn't show up to class, no one would notice. She wanted to give up at the age of ten.

She wasn't just talking about dance. I had heard her say these things before when she made a mistake on her homework or couldn't read as fast as her friends. "Mama, there is something wrong with me. Everyone else can do it, but I can't."

I didn't say a thing. I moved next to her on the couch and lifted her narrow shoulders onto my lap. She was wearing purple leggings and a blue t-shirt with "Dreams come true" written in sequins. I knew the feeling of not being good enough. It woke me up at three in the morning with the pain of how I swallowed what I wanted to say in an important meeting, or how I was falling short of everyone's expectations at home. But I had long ago learned to hide that pain and to keep driving forward believing that if I kept moving, no one would notice that I was not the leader or the mother that people were counting on. I would only slow down when I got sick. Then I got so sick from the stress that I had to face my fear of letting everyone down, or die. There is nothing benign about believing we have to earn our value on the planet.

The opposite of joy is not sadness; it's perfectionism.

I don't mean the have-to-have-your-nails-done-to-go-to-the-store kind of perfectionism. What concerns me is the kind of perfectionism that says, "I'm so sure I'm going to be terrible, I won't even try." Or the kind that researcher Brené Brown points out as our constant drive to earn approval and to "please. perform. perfect. prove."

The world doesn't need us to be perfect; it just needs us to contribute to the common good.

I listened to my daughter cry some more. It made me very uncomfortable to do nothing but hold her. I had to trust that she would find her way, even when the world was constantly telling her that to be average is to be worthless, and if you're not the top, you are the bottom. Fear said, "You are a bad mother. Do something, anything. Make her suffering stop."

I know Fear. She and I go way back. She always finds a way to make me worry about something. She comes in my room at night and says crisply in my ear, "You don't have what it takes." When I turned forty, she said, "Poor baby, you could have been somebody. But you missed your chance." Fear has flawless skin and a red pen. She sees a way to improve everything, including this sentence.

"I'm so tired, Mama."

"I know, I am too." I am tired of striving, reaching, improving myself and everyone around me just so we can have an equal shot at belonging. My daughter and I sat on the couch together as the same questions swirled around us, unanswered.

What if I can't keep up with the world's expectations of me? Am I going to do what feels right, or what I have to do to keep my place on this planet?

At seven years old, I know that the ticket to happiness is to make everyone proud. I am the youngest of three children and the only girl. I love my brothers, Jake and Derek. They are big and strong and good at everything. One morning, I am running down the sidewalk, trying to keep up with them. My feet are slapping the cement in red, leather, Mary Jane sandals. We are late for school. My brothers yell over their shoulders, "Keep up!" I am always slow. I am holding them back. My legs hurt. My backpack is heavy. It keeps hitting me in the head as I run.

They disappear through a gate into a stranger's backyard. They have told me about this shortcut to school before, but I've never taken it. I open the gate. I have to make it across the backyard and to the fence. I hear a dog barking. It sounds like a mean dog with a big, low, deep bark. I put my head down and run. The dog barks and barks. I make it to the fence. I feel the chain links dig into my palms. My feet slip as I climb, but I make it to the top. My shirt catches on the top of the fence, but there is no time to loosen it. I hear a screen door open behind me.

The owner is coming out of his house. He is walking toward me, across the yard, yelling, "Hey!" There is not time to untangle my shirt. I swing both legs over and jump. My shirt rips. I land on my feet, then fall forward. My backpack and its weight push my body into the pavement. I taste blood. Then I hear the man yelling, "Hey! You!" I am up, running away from the yard, looking for my brothers. I can see the top of Derek's head as he's running behind the row of parked cars. He is crossing the street now. The light is yellow. I am running so fast my eyes water. I blink back the tears and lean forward. I make fists with my hands to pump my arms the way Jake showed me to. I run faster, faster. I make it before the light turns red, before the cars rush past me. Jake and Derek are standing there, smiling. Jake says, "You're good. You're fast." They are proud of me. I kept up. *I didn't make them late or hold them back. They think I'm fast.* I feel their approval in my heart. I am hooked on their praise.

I am ten years old. I make a club with four other girls. I am small and skinny with a short, bowl haircut, buck teeth, a flat chest, and bony knees. They are tall, long-haired beauties. There are rules: we must play together and only together at recess. We must wear a brand of sweatpants called Cotton Ginny but they must not be the same color as anyone else's in the group. This morning, Natasha breaks the rules.

"She came to school in the same color sweatpants as Sarah. Twice," Ria says accusingly.

"I'm sure she did it on purpose, just so Sarah couldn't wear hers," Carrie adds.

I look down at the painted hopscotch lines on the pavement and throw my rock, then hop quickly from square to square, being careful not to step on the lines. I don't say anything. Fear's voice is loud in my head, "If you speak up, you'll be kicked out too." Natasha is my best friend. We have known each other since kindergarten. Most days after school we sit together on her porch swing, eating Ritz crackers with peanut butter and laughing. Being with Natasha feels like being home.

"Let's vote," suggests Sarah. "Raise your hand if you think Natasha should be kicked out of the club," she says, staring right at me. Then she raises her hand. I look at Carrie and Ria. Their hands are high in the air. I don't remember lifting my arm. I don't remember agreeing. I just want them to stop looking at me. I must have raised my hand because Sarah smiles.

"There. It's unanimous," Sarah says with triumph in her voice.

Natasha is no longer a part of our club. But I am safe. I am still in. *She'll be fine*, I tell myself. I walk home from school just a few sidewalks squares behind Natasha. I hear her crying. I want to go to her, tell her I am sorry, make her peanut-butter Ritz crackers to make everything better, but I don't. I am afraid. I'm with Sarah and Ria and Carrie. I want to belong to the club. Sarah is talking. I have no idea what she is saying. But I throw my head back and laugh loudly anyway. She puts her arm around my shoulder. *I know what that means. She approves. I'm safe.*

When my mom asks me how school was that day, I don't tell her how sad I am or how badly I hurt Natasha. I push my feelings down.

I show my mom my perfect score on my spelling test. "Good for you," she says. Then Dad, who lives across town, comes over to take my brothers and me for the weekend. I overhear my mom tell him about my perfect spelling test and how I beat all the boys in the city track meet. He looks at me proudly. "Is that true?" he asks. I nod. He picks me up and gives me a big bear hug. "I'm so proud of you. You're my star!" He says. *I am Dad's star.* I look at my parents. They are both smiling. I understand something important. Winning track races and earning perfect test scores is the way to make my parents happy. It's as if I've unlocked a secret door. All I have to do is get good grades and run fast; then we'll all be happy, together.

⋰⋱

I am eleven. I am staying at Dad's house for the weekend. I never see Dad just kicking back, the way some fathers do, in front of a Sunday football game on TV. Dad is always in action mode. We grow up on a lake, so sailing is a regular activity on Sundays in the summer. I'm sure we went out on nice, sunny days, but I only remember the slate-gray ones.

One day, when a storm is brewing on the lake, Dad steers the boat *toward* the darkest patches of water because "that's where the wind is." My eyes are glued to the far side of the lake where lightning burns its way from sky to water and the clouds are as black and flat-bottomed as cast-iron skillets. Dad waves happily to the captains steering their boats toward the sheltered harbor, then says to us kids, "Why are they going home when it's just getting good?" To Dad, the storm is far away, and the lake is big. We can always choose a different heading. What is terrifying to me and those other captains is exciting to him.

So, we watch the lightning the way I imagine other families would watch fireworks, except that they would be safe on their checkered blankets on land, while we float in a tiny boat on a big lake between fierce explosions of thunder.

"Hey kids, isn't this a great show?"

Our plastic, yellow slicker hoods nod "yes" in the pouring rain.

"Uh oh," my dad says suddenly.

"What's wrong?" I ask.

"The halyard is stuck on something…Susie! You're the lightest. Come scamper up the mast and untangle the lines," Dad says as if he is saying, "Come throw the ball with me on the lawn."

"What about those dark clouds?" I ask, nervously.

"Plenty of non-threatening sky to the west," he responds.

I am thrilled to be asked. This is a job reserved for my brothers. There's no time to be scared. But it is cold and windy, and I don't really want to go. *The weather will hold. Don't let him down, Susie. He'll never ask again.* Partway up the mast, I can't stop shivering. My teeth knock against each other and rattle my jaw. The wind vibrates the rigging and makes a loud, howling sound. Everything is shaking. Gusts of wind whip my hair across my eyes and I can't see. I'm not that far up, but I can feel the whole boat rock from side to side beneath me. The storm is still far off in the distance, but up here it seems so close I can touch it. Dad's smile is wide as he looks up at me. I know that look. *He is proud of me. I am not delicate or soft. I'm tough.* I'll do anything to win that smile, to earn his love.

"Come on down!" Dad shouts up at me. I can't tell if he is saying that because he doesn't need my help anymore, or because I have failed him. I cling to the mast as the wind pushes and pulls me. I swing way out over the water on one side of the boat, and then way out over the water on the other side. It's time to climb down, but I can't center myself.

I am thirteen and in junior high now. Fortunately, Natasha and I are best friends again. I quit the Cotton Ginny club and showed up at Natasha's house with a box of Ritz crackers and a jar of peanut butter. I apologized and told her that I knew I'd been a jerk. I had let the fear of not fitting in blind me from what really mattered. "I hurt you, and I'm sorry. Being in a popular club is not worth losing you," I told Natasha. She opened the door, and let me in her house. We cried, then laughed, and promised we'd be braver in groups from then on.

Soon, we join the school orchestra; she plays alto saxophone and I play trumpet. We meet three new friends: Teza (flute), Alli (violin), and Jill (trombone). With them, I am relaxed, even funny, totally myself. Around everyone else, I'm nervous and I pretend to be someone I'm not. I steal candy and smokes from the neighborhood store because I want everyone to think I'm cool. But with Alli, Teza, Jill, and Natasha, I am truly brave. I am vulnerable, nerdy, and square. I even read Jane Austen books in front of them. There is no pressure to perform, no expectation to be cool, no need to be perfect.

When I am with these true girlfriends, my inner voice is louder than Fear's voice. That inner voice says, *Write poetry. Return the things you stole. Be there for someone who needs help. Run because you love to run.* There is a power here that feels different than when I am motivated by anxiety or praise. It feels bigger, lighter, and freer.

Together, we are more powerful than alone. We make things happen. We run for student council. When we want to do something for the school, we go into the closet at the back of the cafeteria, our office, and plan it out. When a tornado strikes a small town nearby, we break several school rules to launch a giant fundraiser. We don't put limits on ourselves.

When some friends of ours complain that they are afraid to go into the ravine near the school because of a "violent gang" that hangs out there, we march into the ravine and make friends with the gang. They were not violent. They were just a bunch of boys who looked different and dressed differently. They had been told enough times that they were stupid and didn't belong, so they started to believe it. They stopped going to school. They hung out in the ravine, smoking cigarettes and acting tough. All we had to do was be brave enough to reach out and let them talk. We listened to their stories. And we kept showing up in the ravine, inviting them to be our friends. Eventually, they agreed. Soon the ravine was a place we'd all go to climb trees, play music, and place branches across the creek to build bridges.

The problem is not that things aren't going well. The problem is that I have learned somewhere that more is better. I am doing too many things. I am pulled in so many directions that I forget to pause and recover. I'm a straight-A student, second trumpet in the band, and a star on the track team. I have medals and awards hanging on my bedroom wall: fastest 800-meter run, fastest 1500-meter run, best speech, French prize, valedictorian. Plus, I am chosen to be in the high school musical as an 8th grader. I love it all. I don't want to give up anything. But it's taking a toll. I'm sick a lot.

Already this year I've had bronchitis and now the doctor says I have pneumonia. *Why does my body hate me? None of the other kids get sick. I must be weak.* I am coughing so much my ribs and shoulders ache. "She should stay home from school for at least a week," the doctor says. *I can't miss a day. I'll be so far behind that I'll never catch up.* My mom tucks me into bed. Then she leaves for work. I feel terrible, and I don't mean the coughing. I feel like I am letting everyone down. Plus, I may lose my spot in the play if I miss a practice. When I can't take lying there any longer, I sneak out of the house. My mom comes home from work to find me gone. She searches everywhere, and calls Natasha and Jill. Then she comes to the high school auditorium to take me away. I don't want to go home. I don't want my mom to be here. This is embarrassing. I make myself as small as I can behind a fake rock on stage. But then I give myself away when I have a coughing fit. She walks on stage and drags me home.

"Why didn't you stay in bed?" she asks, worried.

"Mr. P doesn't like the kids who miss rehearsal."

"I can't stop you. Pneumonia can't stop you. What is it going to take to slow you down?" My mom asks.

I don't even understand the question.

⁂

I am sixteen. I love poetry and writing. When I write, I know what I think. I understand how I feel. It brings order to my chaotic mind. I fill pages and pages of my black, hardcover journal with my poems. I also have a crush on a boy. We are studying together at the library. I open my journal and decide to leave it open when I get up to go to the bathroom. *Maybe he'll read my poems and fall in love with my words.* When I return, he is gone. In the margins of one of my poems, he has written, "If there is an original thought in here somewhere, I can't find it." I can't breathe. It feels like someone dropped a bookcase on my chest. *How could I be so stupid?* I stop writing. I will never write again. *He's right. It has all been said before.* I slide the journal in a box and seal the lid, then bring the box to Dad's garage. I place all my other journals in cardboard boxes and stack them on top of one another. *I will never share my personal writing again.*

Then one night I stay awake past one in the morning while my family sleeps. I am working on an essay for history and I keep rewriting the first paragraph. I can't get it right. I don't have anything original to say. Even though I have an A in the class, it feels like I'm going to fail. So I sneak into my brother's room while he is sleeping and open his bottom drawer. I pull out a stack of papers: math tests, science projects, English assignments, and a history essay on the civil rights era. I flip through it to the last page. A teacher has written in bold cursive, "Excellent! A." I see a way to get the grade I need. *You can't do that!* I immediately think. *I wouldn't have to if the teachers weren't working me so hard,* I counter. *It's their fault I'm so tired,* I say to justify my actions. *It's their fault I can't write my own essay. I have no choice.*

I read through my brother's work. It's really good. My teacher will be impressed. And since my brother goes to a private school across town, my public-school teacher will never know.

I walk back upstairs to my room. I start copying the essay, word for word, onto a fresh sheet of paper. Weeks later, my teacher hands back the essay. He has written in all caps, "ORIGINAL! A+" I am elated. Then I remember it's not my work at all. My mood caves. *I am not an original. How do I tell the truth?* I want to roll back the clock, do it over, confess to my teacher. But Fear says, "Then everyone will know the real truth: that you are a fraud." I burn the essay. *No one will know who I really am.*

I am nineteen. I go to school at an elite college in the Northeast. On the outside, I am effortlessly cool. On the inside, I'm convinced that I don't deserve to be here. I don't have what it takes. I believe the college made a mistake, or maybe I got in only because I added geographic diversity. I miss my friends from home: Natasha, Teza, Alli, and Jill. We are scattered across North America at different schools, and my confidence feels scattered too. I learn to read others and assess quickly who they are and what they want. It helps me get into upper level classes and frat parties, but I haven't learned to read myself. I don't know who I am; I am too busy trying to impress others.

The voice of Fear says to me constantly, "You're not enough. Someone else is smarter, faster, prettier, more motivated." I hear it in class, in the hallway of my dormitory, in the locker room. I try to drown out Fear's voice with more accomplishments. I get As. I set records on the track. I lead several clubs.

But I can't seem to write a ten-page paper for a literature class on a subject I love. It's three days overdue. My professor calls me to his office and says, "Everyone has turned theirs in, except you. Have you started?"

"How can I start if I don't know what I'm going to say?"

"Oh, I see. You want it to be perfect even before you begin. Let's try something. Give me the worst five pages you've ever written by Friday."

He can't mean that. But he looks serious.

"I'm serious," he says, reading my mind.

Friday comes and goes. I don't know how to turn in something terrible. My professor calls me back in.

"How about you give me whatever you have by Tuesday."

"All I have are crummy sentences and quotations."

"Great. I'll take those."

I know what my professor is trying to do, but I can't turn in something average. I think, *It's so late, it needs to be extraordinary.* So, I stay up all night and write a paper that is ten pages longer than the assignment, with a dozen extra references. I turn it in, finally, ten days late. Then I'm sick for a week. I assume that everyone's college experience is like this: all-nighters, followed by sickness, followed by all-nighters, followed by sickness. In my world, it is.

On the upside, I have a boyfriend. He is older than me. I look up to him and want to please him. The first time we have sex, I leave my shirt on. I'm ashamed of my flat chest. *He'll be disappointed.* I move like a gymnast to dazzle him with my flexibility. I don't notice that he is trying to slow me down. I am so busy trying to entertain him, I feel like I've got a top hat and cane. He doesn't ask what I like and don't like, but it doesn't matter. I have no idea. I feel empty inside.

When things aren't working between us, I can't bring myself to break up with him. Fear says, "How can you end it? You started it. You are selfish and cruel." Instead of telling him that my feelings have changed, I avoid him. Then I cheat on him. The relationship ends. I am devastated. But I am also relieved. Then I feel bad for feeling relieved. I move so fast into the next relationship I don't take the time to think about who I am and what I want. *I just want someone to hold me. I just want the emptiness I feel to go away.*

I am twenty-one. It's a sticky, hot afternoon, and I have one more sales call to go. I graduated from college and I am selling knives so I can go hike the Pacific Coast Trail. Yesterday, I drove one-hundred miles to sell a bagel spreader. Today, I knock on the heavy door of a three-storied, red-bricked home to sell a carving set. This address was given to me by a friend of a friend. A woman dressed in a tailored gray blazer and skirt lets me in. She is short, but towers over me with her suspicious stare and firm handshake. I ask for a tomato and a penny. I dice the tomato then decoratively coil the penny into a pig's tail with our best-selling kitchen scissors. I look down at my notes for the final question, "So, Mrs. Bartlett, do you want the Classic Carving Set with scissors or the Holiday Carving Set with a tomato trimmer?" Then I stop. I know that name. I suddenly know exactly where I am. This is Noah Bartlett's kitchen and I am pitching his mom a carving set. Years ago, Noah and I shared first prize in a schoolwide essay contest.

Noah's mom suddenly recognizes me, too. She looks at me hard and does not mince words, "Noah is in China. He is writing his second book with his Princeton professor. And you…" She pauses and looks at me with a mix of pity and judgment, "What are you doing?"

"Selling knives. So I can go hiking," I stammer.

"Don't you have any ambition?"

The words sting. *Everyone is doing more and succeeding more than I am. If I am as smart as those elementary school teachers thought, why am I working a job that has me driving a hundred miles to sell a bagel spreader? I'm a disappointment to my parents.* I get out of that house as quickly as I can. Then I quit. I hike a long section of the Pacific Coast Trail, but only after I polish my resume and send out fifty applications for "real" jobs. *I am going to change the world.*

I become a teacher, like my mother, my aunt, my grandmother, and my great-grandmother before me. I love my job. I like the look of concentration on my students' faces. I love clean chalkboards and the smell of sharpened pencils. I imagine all the discoveries my students and I are going to make as we read and explore new ideas. But I am surprised by the question I hear most often. My students ask, "Is this right?" as in, "Is this answer right?" or "Did I do this essay right?" They don't ask questions born from curiosity, but from fear. I understand my students' desire to please and to perform too well. But that doesn't help my students who collapse on my couch in anxious tears. They say, "I'm so tired of needing perfect grades, perfect test scores, and the perfect body."

How do we banish the idea that we have to be perfect before we begin?

2

I meet my future husband in the middle of the Pacific Ocean. It is a clear, calm day. I am the only beginner among expert kayakers going to Anacapa Island, thirteen miles off Santa Barbara, California.

What am I doing here? I left a great teaching career to take a job working for a famous mountaineer, Rick Ridgeway. I met him and his wonderful wife, Jennifer, when I was teaching their oldest daughter. I help Rick develop book ideas and film proposals for *National Geographic* and the Discovery Channel. He works project-to-project, never knowing when the next paycheck might roll in. This uncertainty makes me anxious, which makes ours a good working partnership. He goes on risky adventures, while I stay back in the office and secure the next contract.

One week, Rick asks to see me. He doesn't like meetings, at least not the conference-room kind. He prefers "floating meetings." This means that we get together at the local surf break and talk business. I zip up my wetsuit and wax my board nervously, because the waves are a fair size today and I don't know how I'll be able to keep up with Rick, much less concentrate on agenda items, as the waves crash around us. But I can't let him down.

I walk to the water's edge and step reluctantly into the freezing, roiling ocean. Rick surfs powerfully, while I flail on my giant longboard. Between waves, we float on our boards and I listen to Rick's latest idea for an expedition, a book, and for conserving more wild spaces around the world. We discuss plans and logistics. He is energized and tossing tasks at me quickly. *How am I going to remember all these details?* I wish there was a way to keep a pen and notebook in my wetsuit. As I am daydreaming about waterproof paper, Rick surprises me with a request.

"I want you to interview someone for my next book who will only be in the country for five days." Rick says.

"So you want me to meet him at the airport?" I guess.

"No, the whole time he'll be in a kayak. I want you to paddle across open ocean with him. Have you ever been in a sea kayak?" Rick asks.

"No," I say.

"Well, want to try something new? What do you say?"

Before I can answer, Yvon Chouinard paddles his surfboard next to us. Rick and Yvon are old friends, having climbed together in Tibet, Bhutan, Chile, and Argentina, among other places. Yvon and his wife, Melinda, started the Patagonia clothing company just a block from here. Yvon often surfs at this local break, and sometimes joins us.

Now there are two adventure legends looking at me, waiting for my answer. *How can I say no?* I remember one of Rick's favorite sayings, "Commit. Then figure it out."

"Well, if you think I can do it..."

Yvon is a man of few words. He sits back, pivots his board to catch a wave, and looks at us.

"Enough talk. C'mon, let's surf," Yvon says with a mischievous grin. He pops up on the wave and glides effortlessly down its liquid-green face. Rick stares at me, waiting.

"Yes?" I say to Rick, more of a question than a statement. It's enough for him. He gives me a big, approving smile, then spins on his board to catch the next wave.

How hard can it be? I think to myself.

Turns out, pretty hard. There is a big difference between surfing near shore and heading out into open ocean in a narrow kayak. One week later, I am floating in a vast sea where there are sharks, shipping lanes, unpredictable winds, and massive waves to worry about. To make matters worse, the man Rick wants me to interview refuses to talk until we reach the island, twelve miles into the Pacific. *Now I have to go. There is no turning back.*

Paddling the kayak feels easy, but I am not going very far or fast. Still, I feel good. I'm pulling it off; no one in our group knows I am a rookie, I think.

"You're holding the paddle upside down," says a gentle voice.

The voice belongs to a guy with curly brown hair and a long beard. He slides his kayak next to mine, shows me how to hold the paddle, and doesn't make a big scene.

"I'm Kurt," he says. "I'm one of the kayak guides your interviewee hired; I'm here to help the group navigate the shipping lanes and shark-y areas."

"Oh. Is this where they found the girl's body last year, eaten by a shark?"

"Well, they're not sure that the shark killed the girl. It may have snacked on her after the fact," says Kurt. As if that makes it all better.

I start paddling fast toward the island. I have a sudden urge to reach land.

"Let's take a compass bearing first, Speedy," Kurt jokes.

Meanwhile, the man I am supposed to be interviewing is far ahead of us, working with another guide. There's no chance we can talk now.

I realize that there is no way for me to reach him or land for several hours. Luckily, Kurt is here and wants to talk.

"So is it true? Are the poles really going to switch?" I say out of the blue. I read once that the Earth's magnetic field inexplicably reverses itself sometimes, so that the north magnetic pole becomes the south.

I am hoping that someone who can navigate with a compass can reassure me about this event.

"Oh yeah. Pretty soon now," Kurt says, without hesitation.

"But if we lose north, what will we set our compasses to?"

"Well, we may have to look south to find north," he says with a mix of wonder and jest. A flock of pelicans glides by us, an inch from the sea's surface, somehow never dipping their blue-gray wingtips in the ocean.

"Birds and whales migrate thousands of miles and they don't rely on any one thing," he continues. "They've blindfolded birds and attached magnets to their heads to scramble the magnetic field. The birds always make it home," Kurt says.

"So they have something like a deeper, internal compass to guide them?" I ask.

"It seems like it. Or just multiple ways to locate themselves. Whales navigate through the arctic by bouncing calls off the undersides of the ice and listening for the echoes."

"How do you know all this stuff?" I ask.

"I read maybe more than I should," he smirks. "You know what I think about?" asks Kurt.

I shake my head.

"If the word compass means 'all that surrounds us,' then maybe we need to wander. We need to get lost to widen our perspective. Maybe it's not about adjusting our instruments, but adjusting the way we look at things."

I am falling for this boy's mind. We paddle and talk easily. Four hours later, we land on a rocky beach on Anacapa Island, not much more than a seagull-infested rock in the ocean. After lunch, Kurt and his friend Scott hitch a ride on a ferry back to the mainland and leave us alone on Anacapa Island.

"Sorry, we have to get back to guide another group," says Scott.

After they leave, I realize that I have no idea what Kurt's last name is. I am sure I'll never see him again.

Two days later, after I've finished the interviews, we paddle home. When I get back to my old, red, Subaru station wagon, there is bird shit all over the hood. There is also a parking ticket on the windshield. I rip the ticket off the window. On the back side of the ticket, a phone number is scribbled in black Sharpie with the words, "Let's go for a walk in Cold Spring canyon!" It is signed, "Kurt." The invitation makes me feel curious, but vulnerable. *Who goes for a walk with a stranger in a canyon?* Then I remember how gentle Kurt was on the water, and how kind.

On my first date with Kurt, I sit near the creek and read poetry while he scrambles up rock faces easily, lightly, looking for birds. He tells great stories of which he is never the center of attention. We go on a few more hikes together. We lose track of time, identifying animal tracks, plants, and bird songs. Then one day, he cuts his hair and shaves the beard off and it is as if I am seeing him for the first time. He has gorgeous eyes. We find shade in secret caves and discover how well our bodies fit together.

"Here, I made you something," Kurt says. He hands me a brown, woven bracelet.

"What is it made out of?" I ask.

"Dogbane fibers. They are super strong. Want me to tie it on your wrist?"

"Sure," I say. I find it exotic to be with someone who can make jewelry out of weeds.

It is dangerous falling in love with Kurt. On the one hand, he is brilliant, honest, and hilarious. On the other hand, he doesn't seem to own shoes. For as long as I can remember, I have had a list of what makes the perfect partner. Fear says, "How can you fall for someone who doesn't satisfy the requirements on that list?"

My list:

- 6'5
- Canadian
- Pacifist
- Ivy-League graduate
- Clean-shaven
- Outgoing, a people person
- Loves poetry
- Runs faster than me
- Goal-driven
- Ambitious

Kurt, when I meet him:

- 5'11
- American
- Ex-marine
- State-school graduate
- Shaggy, old-growth beard

- Likes animals more than people
- Doesn't read poetry
- Hates to run, except on all fours like an animal
- Lives in a tent
- Never wears shoes

Surrendering to the magnetic pull of this relationship is not comfortable for me. To trust the relationship, I have to let go of control and expectations. The more I trust, the more I gain. We go on adventures together, sometimes with maps and compasses, sometimes without. I like myself when I am with him; I am relaxed, confident, and creative. I am not worried about being perfect. With him, I feel like I belong.

I throw my perfect partner list into the wind and watch it blow away. Fear babbles incessantly in my head, giving me reasons why I shouldn't, but I do it anyway. It feels reckless. But it also feels like I am being held. I remember this feeling from when I was very young, leaping into a cold lake. Terrifying and delicious. But I didn't drown. The water held me.

I am used to spending my mental energy worrying. *Is this right? What if this is terribly wrong and I should be with someone else?* But now, instead of worrying, I daydream about our next adventure together. With Kurt, my voice has powerful ease. I say what I feel like saying. I don't feel the usual societal pressure to be cute or witty. I also don't feel like I have to prove that I am not needy. I've even stopped checking myself in the mirror to see how I look. It feels like I'm peeling off layers of caution and prudence and finding my skin underneath, young and shining.

3

We are married under two oak trees, not far from the ocean where we met. But we soon move to Arizona, then to Vermont, and the changes rattle me. With each goodbye to friends and family, I feel like part of me is left behind. *At least we have each other*, I think. But I am not convinced that it is enough. My strong, independent voice feels shaky and weak. I keep looking for a script. I wonder how to act when we are broke and he is unemployed. *What would a good wife say now?*

There is no time for adventures. There is no time for poetry or long walks. He commutes an hour and a half each way to graduate school. I have a job with a lot of responsibility, and I work sixty-hour weeks. At thirty years old, I am part of a small team, running a residential school with motivated teenagers from across the country. I keep wondering when the grown-ups will show up to take over. *Can I really be in charge? If something happens to one of the students, it's on me.* I feel that pressure with every class I teach, every meeting I run, and every time we let the students explore the woods alone.

My colleagues are like the A-team of teachers. I am the new kid. They are brilliant, experienced, and unconventional. They quote Thoreau and T.S. Eliot over breakfast. They know how to play the accordion and solve page-long mathematical equations. I feel simultaneously giddy and anxious among them. They say things about other schools and other leaders that are not generous. It scares me. *Is that how they talk about me behind my back?* I don't feel smart. I don't feel like I deserve to be here. I feel like someone is going to knock on the door any minute and say, "We've found you out. Come with us. You don't belong here."

I stay up late grading papers, preparing for classes and board meetings, then answering emails from anxious parents to prove my worth. The voice in my head is critical. It sounds like a picky principal: "Susie is awkward and keeps missing the point. Her students like her, but they would respect her more if she knew the material better. As an administrator, she fails to consider all of the details. Susie needs to prepare more, manage her time better, and be more professional. She lacks the raw material to be a true leader."

I miss my brothers, who always know what to do. I miss my girlfriends, the ones I call my sisters, who pick me up, brush the dirt off, and help me get back in the arena. We live in rural Vermont now, and they are all back in Canada, at least ten hours away.

I cannot remember the last time I did something for myself. I feel the walls pressing in on me in our apartment. *It's too much. I am not enough.* I shut down the computer and walk outside. Kurt and all of the students are asleep.

Kurt finds me standing under the stars in just a t-shirt on a cold, October night.

"Come to bed," he urges.

"I've got to get out of here," I say in response.

"Maybe you should put some pants on first," Kurt teases gently.

The next day, I check myself into a motel. *I'm going away. I can't keep up.* "Don't tell anyone," I beg Kurt. My colleagues and students can't know I am falling apart. I don't remember how I got to the motel. I remember locking the door. I remember lying on my back on green sheets that smell like moth balls and pond water. *What's wrong with me?* I watch TV in a dark room, hours and hours of TV. The commercials with beautiful, perfect women reinforce my feeling that everyone loves their life, except me. *Maybe I don't need to go back. I like it here. Nobody expects me to know the answers here. Maybe I can stay here with the "Golden*

Girls," *eating microwave popcorn forever.* But I do go back. I put on makeup and pretend that I was away on a fun weekend. I stand up to lead the next faculty meeting, saying to myself and anyone who asks, "I'm fine. I'm *fine.*" I had better be, because I find out I'm pregnant.

Four years later, I am still helping to run the residential school in Vermont. Kurt is away at a graduate school conference. We have two children now. The baby is teething and has been crying for forty-five minutes. Our toddler is screaming at me to play with him. "NOW MAMA!" he hollers. He hands me his stuffed cow, the one that moos when you touch it. The baby wails in my arms, her face red. I can't think. There is too much crying and screaming: WHAAAAA. MOOOOO. NOW MAMA! Something inside me snaps, and I explode. I grab the stuffed cow and throw it against the wall, hard. *Make it stop.* I need silence. I want to smash it to pieces. Instead it lands with a thud, but nothing else happens. "Mooooo," it moans. "MOOOOOO," it cries again, louder, it seems. I've succeeded in making it whine *more.* The baby is still crying. My son is also wailing now. I feel suddenly terrible for him. *What have I done?* In angry response, the cow says, "MOOOOOOO." *I need to get out of here. I can't do anything right. I'm not cut out for parenting.*

Kurt walks in the door. I hand him the baby and the broken cow toy. The toddler lifts his arms; he wants to be picked up by his dad. I escape to another room.

I call the number on the crumpled piece of paper. It is for a therapist. A friend recommended her to me years ago, but I never called, because I thought, *Therapy is for broken people with terrible childhoods. I am just a little overwhelmed.* But now I hear a woman's voice on the other end. She sounds kind. She sounds smart. *Can you see me now?* I hear myself ask. I sound like I am begging.

I grab the car keys. I tell Kurt I'm going out. He waves goodbye. I can't tell if he's angry or relieved that I am leaving.

It's early summer in Vermont. As I drive, I feel the thick trees on both sides of the road squeezing in on me. The forest seems dark and unfriendly. And even though my breath is shallow and I can't get air, I roll the window up tightly.

Hilary's office is in her barn, upstairs. The morning light comes in through the giant windows up near the roof and I can see the sky. I want to stay here. I feel like asking her to write me a note, to excuse me from having to go back to the crying and screaming and mooing.

"Do you second-guess yourself?" she asks.

"All the time."

"Give me an example."

"I should not have had children."

"Why do you say that?"

"I'm not good at it. I don't know what to do. I throw their toys at walls. I think about driving across the border and never coming back."

"If a woman feels angry, struggles, and needs quiet to think, then there must be something wrong with her, not with society. Is that what you think?"

"What do you mean by society?"

"Our culture sends a clear message to women: good mothers are calm, loving, and willingly sacrifice themselves for their children. When you fall short of those expectations, the problem isn't that we have created an unattainable myth of mothering, but that you are a failure and broken."

"That's how I feel; I am a failure."

"What do you think when you wake up?"

"Another chance to feel bad all day."

"Do you think you are depressed?"

"I don't know. I have a great husband, great kids, and a great job. How can I be depressed?"

"It's very common."

"Sometimes it's good. Like yesterday, when the rain cleared, the kids and I went on a rainbow and puddle hunt. I felt genuinely happy then."

"Sure. But what keeps you up at night?"

"I feel like I could not survive without my husband or my colleagues, but that they would be totally fine without me. What does that make me?"

"Depressed. Let's get you some medication for now."

"Will that help me get more done?"

"It's not about getting more accomplished; it's about feeling better," she says, laughing a little.

"But if I take the meds to feel better, then that proves that I am a depressed person. And I have no reason to be depressed."

"You don't need a reason. It doesn't matter why you are struggling, it only matters that you are. No amount of working harder will change the chemical imbalance in your brain."

"But that feels like a death sentence, not a solution."

"It's not forever. Things change. You only feel that way because you learned somewhere that you are supposed to be happy all the time. That's a lot of unrealistic pressure."

"But maybe if I did more to be better at mothering, or better at my job, I would feel better, and I would be happy. I wouldn't need meds."

"You don't need to do more, excel more, or accomplish more to be more worthy," she says firmly.

I want to believe her. I hear the truth in what she is saying, but I can't shake the notion that I am broken. I leave her office feeling like I have duct tape on my forehead that labels me as "DEPRESSED."

I am thirty-nine. Ten years into our marriage, Kurt and I are struggling. Maybe it's my depression. But he's the one who seems gloomy. I take my antidepressants every day, but I wonder why I still don't feel happy. Maybe it's just middle-age marriage stuff. I don't know, because no one talks about the difference between normal problems and red-flag warnings. Our relationship is suffering under the weight of stress, children, and money issues. *How do I know this rough patch will pass? What if things never get better?*

One evening, I prepare a big taco dinner for everyone. When I finally sit down, I notice that Kurt is almost done eating. I wait for the kids to leave the table and turn angrily to Kurt.

"Can't you see that I always eat last? Just once I want to sit down and eat first," I say.

"But the food was getting cold," he says sheepishly.

"That's not the point!"

"What is the point?"

"Why can't you just get me?" I snap at him. He opens, then closes his mouth, without saying anything. I don't want to explain that in life, as with this meal, I feel like I put everyone else before me. I want him to put me first without me having to tell him to do so. *Can't he understand that?*

Kurt and I are just too different. He thinks linearly and speaks directly. I think emotionally and speak indirectly. I'm an extravert who feeds off social energy. He is an introvert who prefers to be alone. I should have stuck to my perfect partner list, because all I see now are the cracks and imperfections in Kurt. I want to fix them all.

I bring him to a coffee shop and make him write down his career goals. I think I'm helping, but he feels like I am micromanaging. Things on the surface of our relationship suddenly bother me. I beg him to exercise more, to drink less, and to wear something other than his old blue sweatshirt. I know I'm being shallow, but I can't stop thinking about all the ways he could change for the better. I spend my free time worrying about the future and criticizing him. He ignores me and dives deep into his dissertation. We go to bed at different times. We wake at different times.

One night, I'm up because I'm feeling anxious about our marriage. I notice the way Kurt is sleeping. He lies on his back with his thumbs hooked into the top of his boxers, like a little boy. *It's not his fault,* I think. *We just need a change. A fresh start will save our marriage.*

We move to Colorado. Kurt continues to write his PhD dissertation on black bears. I am offered the position of director in a global education company. I am learning decades worth of material in months. The financials are dizzying. *I should understand them better.* I stay up late sorting through them. When I travel internationally for work, I leave Kurt and the kids behind. There is no time to talk with him about anything other than logistics.

Then there is the stress of risk management. I am responsible for the safety and happiness of hundreds of students around the world. In one quarter, a volcano erupts in Indonesia, there are air strikes in Israel, an Ebola outbreak in Senegal, and a terrorist attack in China. I keep the phone next to my bed; it rings at one in the morning because a student in India may need surgery on her appendix. It rings at three in the morning because we need to re-route a group to avoid kidnappings in Jordan. My journal, which used to be full of poetry, is full of risk management scenarios and strategic plans. I have constant headaches. *I can't keep up.*

Meanwhile, our children grow and so does their number of soccer games, music lessons, dance recitals, and plays. I feel guilty all the time. Fear says, "Good moms don't miss their children's recitals." I don't make it to most soccer games either, because of work. "Every other mom will be there, except you," Fear says, dousing me in shame.

The founder of the company sends me an email blaming me for low enrollment. He says he is not going to offer bonuses this year, and it's my fault. His words feel untrue and make me angry, but they still sting. *I'm not cut out to be the director. I'm failing.* I try to advocate for myself and for the others, detailing our tireless work and successes. But I feel sluggish and inarticulate around him. *Why can't I say the right words to change his mind?* Fear says, "A real leader would know exactly what to say."

Two weeks later, the founder brings me flowers and praises me for my leadership in general. I feel light and successful. *What can I do to win his praise again?* My journal entries shift from strategic plans to strategic ways to please the founder. I hustle and perform for the founder, not for the good of the company. I live and breathe for his approval. I continue to take my antidepressants, but I don't tell anyone that I am struggling inside. I don't even call my girlfriends at home anymore. I imagine that I would sound whiny or needy. They are all so busy; I don't want to be a burden. What would I say? *Hi. Help. I can't remember who I am.*

When the phone rings before dawn because of a crisis on another continent, I can't go back to sleep. I leave Kurt asleep in bed and I put on my running shoes. I follow the trails into the mountains. The rising sun feels like warm hands on my shoulders. *I can breathe.* When I run, I count exhales, not seconds. Time seems to slow down. Deer graze so close to the trail I can almost touch their outstretched ears.

When I run, I know whether I am doing well by the way my body feels, not by what anyone else says. Then comes the moment when all thoughts fall away and all that is left is my wild, animal body. *This is who I am.*

Running on a trail, alone, I am not responsible for the success of a company, or for the success of our marriage. *Nobody needs me. I want to keep running and never stop.*

4

One day, I wake up and try to say good morning to the kids, but I can't. My tongue cramps and no sound comes out. Seconds pass, and my tongue works fine again, but I notice a sharp pain at the back of my head, right at the top of my spine.

"Are you okay?" ask Cole and Hazel when they see me stop and grip the kitchen counter in pain.

"Fine. Fine," I say dismissively, and get back to making their school lunches. When the headaches and tongue cramping occur a few days in a row, I call my doctor. I think, maybe I hurt something when I carried a heavy backpack uphill recently. Maybe a vertebra is out of place.

Dr. Pedersen's walls are a pale brown color with nothing on them but a few diplomas and an anatomical poster of the human body. I sit on the crinkly white paper on the examining table. My doctor is just a few years older than me. Her blonde hair is cut in a professional bob, and she wears a sporty skirt. She always moves quickly, talks quickly, and smiles quickly. I like her; we are not quite friends, but good acquaintances. Our kids are a few grades behind hers at the same neighborhood schools. She asks me about the headaches.

"Any dizziness?"

"No."

"Squeeze my fingers tightly. Now touch your thumb to each forefinger. Can you touch your nose with the tip of your pointer finger? Good. Stand up. Walk in a straight line."

"Is this a sobriety test?" I ask.

"If it were, you'd pass. You're sober. And your brain is fine."

"So why is my tongue cramping?"

"I don't know. But I don't like the sound of that. Let's do an MRI scan of your skull."

A few weeks later, I am back in her office, the headaches and tongue cramps still bothering me.

"The MRI came back clean and normal. You can breathe easy now," my doctor says.

"That's a huge relief. So what is causing the headaches?" I ask.

"How long do you sit in front of a computer each day?" Dr. Pedersen asks.

"At least four hours."

"I'd start there."

I go home and talk to Kurt.

"The doctor says I should get up and move around every twenty minutes," I tell him.

"You were never the sitting down type anyway. I'll build you a standing desk," he offers.

"Could you add a treadmill?"

"Slow down, Seabiscuit. Let's see how the standing part goes first." Then Kurt stays up all night to build me a standing desk. I stay up, too, to keep him company. It's the first time in a while that we do something together, just the two of us. It feels good.

I am grateful for my new desk, but the headaches persist. I see doctors, chiropractors, massage therapists, and physical therapists. Each specialist is convinced that the problem is my pillow. I buy hard pillows, soft pillows, buckwheat pillows, lima-bean-shaped pillows, foam neck pillows, body pillows. There are so many pillows covering our bed that Kurt wonders, "Are the pillows having babies?"

I make an appointment with a highly-recommended massage therapist who works with triathletes and Olympians. After I try massaging my neck and head for a few weeks, my tongue cramping goes away. The headaches persist but are manageable with ibuprofen and the bodywork she gives me. I am convinced it is just stress.

In November 2015, the headaches are manageable enough that I run the New York City marathon to celebrate my friend Sarah's birthday. I am intimidated by Sarah and my other running partners; they are all female champions at this distance, with several of them having run marathons under three hours. Fear now says, "They're real runners. You're an imposter." They run and talk and I do my best to keep up, breathing heavily. "You're holding them back." I listen to Fear and back off. I don't tell them how I feel. Instead, I join them on the short, easy days, and usually skip the intense speed workouts.

We wake up at three thirty in the morning in New York City on a cold, dark, race day. At the start, there are thousands and thousands of people. I lose my friends almost immediately. I am used to running on trails, with almost no one around. *They must be ahead. Don't let them down. Keep up.* I feel frantic and lost. *How will I find them again?* I listen to the rhythm of my own feet. *My pace is too fast; it is unsustainable. But I have to go faster to catch up.* For a few miles, I attach myself to a group of Dutch men in orange shirts who are running strong. I try to stay with them, but I am straining to keep up. I have a headache. *Where are my friends? There's no use. I am way behind.*

At mile twenty, I want to quit. I slow down to a shuffle. *My friends will finish way ahead of me.* An African-American woman on a crowded sidewalk in the Bronx shouts, "I see you, Susie. You CAN do this!" She must be reading my shirt. I had written my name on the front in black Sharpie pen.

"You GO, girl! Do ya hear me, Susie?" Here was a woman who didn't know me at all. I was just a random white lady. My guess was we didn't have much in common, but she saw me struggling and rooted for me. That big-hearted gesture motivated me to finish strong.

I cross the finish line in a decent time with the Bronx woman's strong voice and words of encouragement still ringing in my ears. I want to tell my friends about how much her words meant to me, but they are not at our meeting spot. *Maybe they are already having lunch somewhere?* It turns out they were behind me the whole time. While I ran frantically, convinced that they were faster than me, I missed the fun. They ran a relaxed, easy race and finished together. *Running easy was an option?*

5

Back home in Colorado, the headaches are a part of life. I wake every morning with a heavy pain at the back of my skull, take a couple of ibuprofen, and do yoga to improve my posture before putting in hours in front of the computer. I get a massage as often as I can.

When I ask my massage therapist what she thinks is wrong with me, she says, "I don't tell this to just anyone, but I am often in touch with my clients' spirit guardians and they say things."

"Oh," I say nervously. "What do my spirit guardians say about me?"

"That you were an eagle in your past life. That's why you can run so fast."

"Cool," I manage to say with my face firmly pressed into that round head holder that is like a padded toilet seat. I don't say, though I want to, "Eagles can't run."

"Your guardians say you have a tomahawk wedged in your skull from your past life as a bird."

"That explains it," I say.

"Our job," she says, "is to release the tomahawk."

"That's your job," I feel like saying. "My job is waiting for me."

I hop off the table, write her a check, pop some ibuprofen, and go back to work. There is no time to think about headaches or tomahawks. I have children to feed, meetings to go to, presentations to give, students and guides to care for, emergency evacuations to direct.

After years of this, I finally decide that the stress of my job is not worth the pain of these headaches. I don't renew my contract. It is not an easy decision. I don't want to let anyone down. But the headaches have gotten worse, and I don't know what else to do. The idea is to slow down, work fewer hours, and sit in front of a computer less often. But being out of work means I have more time to worry and doubt myself. Fear doesn't even wait for nighttime anymore to whisper terrible thoughts in my ear; she starts in on me first thing in the morning. "You'll be a bag lady," she sneers, then adds, "Your parents are really disappointed in you."

It also means I have to face the emptiness I feel on the inside. And that is deeply uncomfortable. Instead of facing my feelings, I distract myself with projects. Some people numb with wine or heroin, I numb myself with busyness. I travel to Guatemala to work with Indigenous girls fighting for the right to go to school. I sew costumes for our daughter's ballet performances. I drive my son and his friends to the skate park. I lead a running club for sixty-five elementary school children. Then I find a new job; I manage a social-emotional curriculum aimed at fifty-eight million school children. *How do I say no to any of this?*

When I get home, I am tired and negative. And I don't make the connection that I am stretched too thin. Instead, I focus on Kurt's flaws. *Why doesn't he make the bed? Play with the kids? Take me out on the town? If he did more, I wouldn't be so exhausted.*

My body, meanwhile, seems to be insisting that I am the one who needs to change. It begs me to slow down and do less by giving me a debilitating headache when I speed up or add a project to my plate. But I ignore my body. With a clean MRI, I figure I am just a person who gets headaches. I wake every morning with a throbbing skull, but because I feel better after I run, I continue to train for big races and cope with the pain. Eventually, the headaches go away. Or maybe they don't really go away. Maybe I just get used to them.

∾⅏∾

On my birthday, May 30, 2016, I run a 50-kilometer (31-mile) ultramarathon that begins at an elevation of near 8,000 feet. The "Dirty Thirty" race course is set in a state park in the Rocky Mountains where I live. The course winds up and down on a single-track trail with over 7,250 feet of elevation gain and loss. At twenty-six miles, we climb a 10,000-foot peak before turning around and sprinting the last six miles to the finish, downhill. It's a tough race. This is my third year doing it. I run it for three reasons: (1) the views of the mountains are breathtaking, (2) I like to do something scary on my birthday, and (3) it is a way for me to raise funds for MAIA; Her Infinite Impact, an organization that helps to support the bright, motivated girls I know in Guatemala, to go to school. In 2014, I traveled to Guatemala, looking for ways to close the gender gap in education. Guatemala has the highest level of gender inequality in the Western Hemisphere. I met with Indigenous leaders, Norma and Vilma. After years of being called a "dirty Indian" Norma learned to use her voice to stand up for herself and for young, Indigenous women everywhere. She and Vilma rallied international support to create the MAIA Impact School, the first all-Indigenous, all-female-led school in the Americas.

I wake up at four in the morning to drive to the start with my neighbor and his friend from college, both experienced ultrarunners. It's not even forty degrees outside. I am cold and nervous. I am seriously undertrained. I also have a headache. I consider dropping out, but then I think about the girls in Guatemala. *I can't let them down.* I fill out the emergency information on the back of my race number, and put Kurt down as my contact should I collapse midway through the race. I've run in countless races, but I've never actually bothered to fill out this emergency form. This time, something tells me I might need help. I brush off the thought, but write Kurt's number down legibly anyway.

The gun goes off at dawn. At mile three, I drop my water bottle on the trail. The nozzle fills with mud and clogs it. From that point on, every time I sip water, I get only dirt.

At mile seven, I have to stop running. My legs are cramping, I have a headache, and the altitude is getting to me. I feel like I am breathing through a snorkel. I walk. *C'mon Susie. It's only mile seven!* A steady stream of runners pass me. I feel defeated. I walk with my head down. *I didn't train enough. I'll quit as soon as I make it to a road.*

I hear the cheers from the aid station through the next patch of trees. Then two volunteers hand me water, oranges, fig bars, and M&Ms. I shove the candy in my mouth, wash it down with water, and suddenly I feel better. I check in with my body: no leg cramps, no headache, no pain anywhere. I decide to keep going. *Lift your eyes. It's beautiful here.* And it is. I listen to the Aspen trees quake, the rivers rush over smooth stones, and sensation the sun on my face. I feel strong and light. I also decide to dedicate each mile to someone, mostly the young women I know best in Guatemala: Norma, Vilma, Irma, and Jeronima. This helps me to keep going.

At mile twenty-six, the point at which marathoners can see the finish line, the race course takes a left turn to climb Windy Peak, a 10,000-foot summit that usually strips the oxygen from my legs one switchback at a time. But this time I feel light and strong. I dedicate this section to Kurt.

In places, the mountain is so steep I have to use tree trunks like ladder rungs to pull myself up the trail. Where there are no trees, I slide backwards on the steep slope that moves with each step. I consider giving up for good. Then, I imagine Kurt's face in my mind, and I start to cry. I see through his trivial imperfections and remember why

I fell for him. Maybe it's the endorphins. But it feels deeper and more real than a case of lightheadedness. Everything that isn't important falls away. What is left is love. Suddenly, the loose scree feels solid and the mountain seems less steep.

When I reach the top, I am euphoric. I ask the course official to snap a photo of me leaping into the sky. I can't believe I am here and have made it this far today. It's as if running to the summit has lifted me out of a dark cloud of negativity. It's clear to me that I could never have made it this far without Kurt. It's also clear that I want to move forward with him, no matter how different we are. But right now, I still have six miles to go, running down a sheer mountainside.

I realize that I haven't seen many women go by. *Maybe I'm doing better than I think.* I turn and run downhill, but my legs feel like jello. I'm not sure my muscles can last much longer at this altitude. Still, I notice that if I lean forward, like I am daring the mountain to knock me down, my legs find strength under me. I run by feeling, not thinking. *I feel brave. I feel indomitable.*

I see our kids not far from the finish line. Cole and Hazel jump up and down, shouting, "You can do it, Mama!" Then they run alongside me in their little sandals. We cross the line together. I end up finishing as the first woman in the masters division, a competitive age group in Boulder, Colorado. I am shocked and elated. There were many moments in the race when I wanted to quit because I was convinced I was doing so poorly. Turns out, that was all in my mind. *How many times have I been doing well in my life and just assumed that I was failing?*

I lie down in the rushing creek and Kurt brings me a beer. I tell him about how I dedicated the hardest section to him, and he chuckles. He can't help but make a joke. He pretends to be me, and quips: *"Let me see, who makes my life really difficult and yet I endure anyway? I know! Kurt!"* It feels good to sit side-by-side with him in the river, laughing. We let the current wash over us, and we link arms to hold steady against its pull. Together, we make a good anchor.

Thirty-one miles. Twenty-seven creek crossings. Two serious mountain passes. All behind me now. I feel alive, vigorous, and capable of anything.

Two weeks later, I learn that I have between three and five months to live.

The Opposite of Joy is Perfectionism

We are born with only two fears: the fears of falling and of loud noises. As we grow, our fears grow too. We worry about what we might lose instead of what we might gain. We don't think of ourselves as perfectionists, but we're scared to try things that don't guarantee us a positive outcome. As Brené Brown writes in *Dare to Lead*, "Healthy striving is self-focused. How can I improve? Perfectionism is other-focused: What will people think? Perfectionism is a hustle." The good news is that once we identify our kind of perfectionism, and see it as a lousy shield between us and the world, we can drop it. It helps to remember that our innate selves are brave. When we take risks, we actually start to feel *more* like ourselves.

To stem the tide of perfectionism and the anxious feelings that go with it:

- *Remember when you were ten years old.* What did you love to do? Let those memories inform your true comfort zone and develop a mindset of being born brave.

- *Flip (off) the inner critic.* By flipping each negative thought to a positive one, we can catch those unkind thoughts faster, recover quicker, and spin out less often. "I'm not doing enough" becomes "I am enough." "My body is too heavy" becomes "My thoughts are heavy; I am light."

- *Make risk-taking so normal, it is boring.* Take risks early and often. Take your writing public. Say no to someone powerful. Try a new skill. Share your true feelings about something. Face conflict. Notice how the ground doesn't fall away.

- *Feel the fear and do it anyway.* I believe that we are capable of so much more than we think. But we're scared as sh** sometimes.

Fear is just part of the process of doing something new. We need to feel it, drop stories attached to it, and step through it.

- *Notice how far you've come, not where everyone else is standing.* A life of comparing and competing has consequences. Instead of making us stronger, it can cause us to feel anxious. I love when writer Anne Lamott says, "Never compare your insides with everyone else's outsides." Take the long view; trust that you are exactly where you need to be now, becoming who you are meant to be, at your own pace.

- *Keep a record of moments when you survived discomfort.* Maybe you remember the soreness you felt when you first got braces. Or the devastation you felt when your first love dissolved. Return to what helped you get through tough times to remember your inner resiliency.

- *Build a community that celebrates progress, not perfectionism.* Ask yourself, then your colleagues and friends, "Where did you make progress today?" instead of "What did you get done today?" Host "no-talent" shows and "story slams," where people are invited to share stories that don't leave out the struggle and failure. Celebrate persistence, vulnerability, and contributions to the common good, not merely accomplishments.

PART II

BRAVE OVER PERFECT

6

"First, you'll lose your voice. Then your ability to breathe," says Dr. Levin, lifting his glasses to the top of his head to look at me and Kurt directly. He says these words in the same matter-of-fact tone that a waiter might say, "First your salad will arrive. Then you'll get your steak." He takes a plastic model of a skull down from a shelf in the cramped examination room and points at its waxy yellow bones and purple plastic arteries, giving a lecture on the brainstem's function. I recognize that it is a human skull, but I have no idea what he is saying. My mind drifts to my heart. *Is it beating?* Then to my lungs. *Can I still take a breath?*

How did I get here? Two weeks after running the ultramarathon, I wake up with a bad headache. I am not surprised. I am used to this throbbing discomfort, and I was also up late with girlfriends, drinking wine. But this feels sharper than the dull fogginess of a hangover. And it's accompanied by an electric pain radiating down my right arm. I have not felt this before. I manage to drive the kids to their summer day camps. On the way home, while stopped at a traffic light, I suddenly feel nauseated. I open the car door and throw up on the white line in the middle of the road. Something is not right, but I have no idea what is wrong. I wipe my mouth, drive home, and call my friend Sarah. She offers to take me to the doctor. Dr. Pedersen orders a new round of MRIs of my head and neck, and that's how I end up in this neurosurgeon's office.

"We can't know what kind of tumor this is for sure until we get a piece of it, but it's rare and aggressive. It has wrapped itself like a boa constrictor around your brainstem. The brainstem controls your heart, your lungs, everything you need to survive," says Dr. Levin.

We found this doctor online by typing "skull base tumor neurologist Colorado" into Google and seeing only a few names show up on the computer screen. Dr. Levin fit us in quickly after receiving the scans of my skull in the mail. He is a tall, fit man in his sixties with white hair and thick glasses. He is wearing a purple button-down shirt with no tie and has a habit of moving his glasses off his face when he speaks.

At forty-five years old, I have been, up until this moment, medically "boring." No health or genetic history of any kind. Previous conditions: none. Previous surgeries: wisdom teeth removal. I am a champion runner who competes in ultramarathons. *What is he saying?*

"The tumor has engulfed every major artery, nerve, and ligament moving from your brain down your spine. It's hard to tell, but it also looks like it has eaten the bones at the top of your spine, including the peg that holds your head on your neck." Again, he lifts his glasses off his nose to look at me. He is trying to see if I understand. I just stare at the skull in his hands. It's a lot to digest.

"Are you saying that the only thing holding my head on my body right now is this tumor?"

"Possibly."

"Can you remove it without damaging the brainstem or knocking my head off?"

"It will require two, maybe three operations to remove what we can of the tumor. There are, of course, serious risks," he says. Dr. Levin looks at us with an apologetic expression, then puts the skull back on the shelf.

"What kind of risks?" Kurt asks.

"Death. Paralysis. Brain deficits. Inability to eat or breathe on her own," he lists.

"And what if we don't operate?" I ask.

"I give you three, maybe five months to live." I look at the surgeon's kind face, but there is no sign that he is joking. Kurt puts his notebook down and gently reaches for my hand.

Fear tightens every muscle in my body. Fear says, *"Your children will grow up without a mother."* I think of Hazel, our daughter. How do we tell her? At ten years old, she still loves magic, fairies, and mermaids. Her favorite toy is a purple fairy that uses leaves to heal the sick or the broken. I feel rage toward the doctor. I want to shout, "You tell Hazel that her mother is dying. Then tell her that the leaf-bandages won't be enough." But I don't. My mouth opens and closes, but no sound comes out.

Then I think of Cole, her older brother. He has always built forts and spaceships and skate ramps. I imagine him now at twelve, trying to be strong for me, for his sister, for his father. I can picture him silently building a fort in our home. But what can he build that would protect any of us?

Now, in this neurosurgeon's tiny examining room, Fear is the loudest voice in my head. Her microphone is working just fine. She repeats, "Your children will grow up without a mother."

⁂

"How does your voice feel now?" Dr. Levin asks, "Are you able to use it whenever you want?"

"Yes," I say, but the question hangs in the air for a moment.

Usually, when the topic of using your voice is mentioned, it's about permission. I feel lucky to be born in a time and place where I am free to speak out. But that doesn't mean I have always known how to find my voice and how to use it to author my life. *Is it an accident that the tumor is sitting on my vocal cords and the part of the brain where some say fear is born?* I stare at the doctor's computer screen with the black and white images of my skull. The area inside my head is black except for this large, white growth, shaped like a storm cloud, pushing into the dark spaces around my brain, tongue, and vocal cords. *I will die young and without a voice.*

"Go home. Take time to consider the operations. But not too much time. This tumor needs immediate attention," says Dr. Levin.

"What kind of tumor is it?" I ask.

"I don't know. It looks like a chordoma or a chondroma, but there is no way to know exactly until they have a good look at it during surgery."

"Is it benign? Malignant?"

"It's aggressive; that's all we know."

"What about a biopsy?"

"I don't recommend it. The tumor is too close to every major nerve and artery to perform any extra surgeries."

"So we just wait and see?"

"You live your life. The tumor has to come out. And when it does, we'll know what it is. There's no use guessing now."

The doctor shakes our hands goodbye. He has a crowded waiting room of people expecting him.

Once he's gone, I rock back and forth on the examining table. Then I cry, grunt, and growl while Kurt holds me tight. I make animal sounds that I don't recognize. *When will I lose my voice?*

I am used to making things happen, using my strong will to push beyond obstacles. I am comfortable sprinting up mountain passes, throwing up from dehydration, running with a dislocated shoulder. But now, there is nothing I can do to push through or change my situation. I have no idea how to behave. I am not even sure who I am.

When was the last time I genuinely used my voice? What I mean is, *When did I last say what I felt, not what I thought others wanted to hear?* I think back to the Monday before I got the news about the tumor. I woke up with a bad headache and I felt raw and cranky. In the kitchen, Kurt cracked eggs into a hot cast-iron skillet. Instead of saying *I feel terrible*, I used my voice to say, "Should you really be having two fried eggs for breakfast *again?*" Kurt looked at me, hurt. Later, a neighbor asked if I would be the recycling coordinator for the neighborhood. I wanted to say "No, thanks," but I said, "Yes, of course!" I didn't want to disappoint him. At work, I was sprinting to meet an unrealistic timeline. My colleagues asked, "How's the project going?" I didn't want them to think that I couldn't handle it on my own, so instead of asking for help, I said, "It's going great." When I finally arrived at home and felt the buildup of not using my voice all day, I unleashed on my children. They were quietly playing a video game. I didn't say hello or ask, "What are you playing?" I used my voice to scream, "Get off that f*&?#@!! screen." They left the room, sobbing.

Now, using my voice is a matter of life or death. What if this tumor moved into the place near my vocal cords because the area seemed abandoned? The question in my mind went from, *When will I lose my voice?* to *When did I let it go?*

I like to talk. But rarely do I say what I mean. For too long, my voice has said what I think a good leader, a good wife, and a good mother *should* say. I am used to saying someone else's lines because I don't trust my own voice to be inspiring enough, calm enough, or wise enough. *How could I possibly know what to say?*

It wasn't always like this. When I was a little girl, I said what I wanted to say without worrying about how it might sound. I sang loudly on the front steps, into my broom-handle microphone, to any passersby who would listen. I read original poetry at family gatherings. I wrote long letters to Santa listing exactly what I wanted and where he might find the Play-Doh Fuzzy Pumper Barber and Beauty Shop on sale. I also did what I felt like doing. If I had an urge to climb a tree and sit in it all day, pretending to be a squirrel, I didn't second-guess myself. I got to work collecting nuts. If I didn't want to sit next to my nicotine-breath grandmother on the couch, I didn't. I sat on the floor at her feet and listened to her hilarious stories. I knew my yeses from my nos. I had boundaries and convictions; I knew where I began and others ended. But lately, I have lost touch with who I am, what I want, and what my true voice sounds like.

Time is running out. I am determined; I will say what I feel and knock this hobo tumor right out of my brainstem railcar. Maybe it will send a message to the tumor saying, *Sorry. No Vacancy: this space is occupied and home to a powerful, wild voice that cannot be silenced.*

"Well, what do you want to do now?" Kurt asks. We are sitting in our gray car in a sea of gray cars in the parking lot of the hospital in Denver, Colorado after seeing Dr. Levin.

"Drive to the mountains," I say, without hesitating. It feels different; it feels good to listen to my inner voice and discover what appeals to me and what doesn't right now. I don't want to be around people. I want to lean against a rock and sit under a big, ponderosa pine. I want to be held, but I also feel like pulling away. I want to touch something solid, like a mountain.

"What do we tell the kids?" I ask. I picture their sweet faces: our twelve-year-old red-haired boy and our ten-year-old girl with freckles on her nose. Then I burst into tears.

"I don't know. But we'll figure it out," Kurt says. He puts the car in drive.

We go to the mountains. We sit among deep, red rocks, overlooking the plains and don't say anything for a long time. Then Kurt says,

"Happy sixteenth anniversary."

"Well that's totally unfair," I say.

"You mean," Kurt says, "discovering you have a massive tumor is fine, but finding out that you have a tumor on our anniversary is totally unfair?"

"Exactly," I say. And finally, I let him hug me tight. Then I cry. I cry for how good I have it. I cry because I don't want it to end so soon. I cry because I am scared. *How are we going to do this? How will the kids handle the news?* Crying feels like a release. But it also feels like accepting this tumor and I don't want to accept it as real. I want to dry my tears and go home and find out tomorrow that this was all a dream.

If I cry, it feels real. If I accept it, am I giving in? Am I giving up? *I don't like giving up.* I like winning. I like being in charge. Right now, I am so obviously not in charge of my life. *I* would never have done this to any woman, and certainly not a mother. *Never.*

"Let's renew our vows," I say, suddenly. I'm not sure why. But it comes from deep inside me.

"Here? Now?"

"Yes. You go first," I say, teasingly. But he doesn't hesitate.

"I take you, Susie, to be my wife, to have and to hold, in sickness and in health, until death do us part. And…" he pauses to make sure I am looking at him.

"If I could switch places with you right now and be the one with this diagnosis, I would." Kurt says the words with such love and certainty that I cry again. I bawl. I thought that this news might make him want to pack his bags and leave. Now I realize that I wanted to renew our vows because I wanted to make sure he wasn't going to run away. But he has no intention of leaving me. My nose is running, but I don't want to let go of his hands. So I lean over and wipe my nose on his jacket sleeve. He laughs. Then it is my turn.

"I take you, Kurt, to be my husband, to have and to hold, in sickness and in health, until death do us part. This is out of our hands, but so was finding each other, and that has turned out even better than I could have imagined." It feels good to say. *When was the last time I told Kurt how much I truly love him?* The sun washes Kurt's face and the rocks behind him in apricot-stained light. *Why don't I tell him every day how much I love him?*

I think I am ready to face the kids, but it is so beautiful outside that the pain of dying young washes over me. I burst out in tears, "I want to stay!" And what I mean is, I want to stay on this earth. I want to stay being Kurt's wife. I want to stay as the mother of our children. I want to stay to watch the light soak these mountains in a red rinse until I have gray hair and can no longer get up out of my rocking chair to turn away from rock and sky and sun. My feet refuse to move from where I stand. Then Kurt gently guides me by the hand, back to the car.

The drive home is a blur. We compose an email to our families on scrap paper we find in the glove box. Then we call our parents—mine first. My mom says confidently, "You've got this. You've been training your whole life for big challenges." My dad, a lover of slogans, tells me to be "strong like a streetcar!" Next, we call Kurt's parents. They sign off the same way they always do, "Love you. Our bags are packed if you need help." Talking to both sets of parents is hard. You never want to worry your parents, and I can tell that they are very worried. I recognize how difficult it must be to be a parent when your child is really sick. I feel strangely grateful that I am the one with the tumor.

When we arrive home, it is cool outside and the children are silly and playful. It doesn't feel right to squash their joy with news that they can't do anything about. Kurt and I delay telling them. We look in the fridge to figure out what to make for dinner. We serve leftover pasta, and a single green pepper as "salad." After dinner, we sit on our front porch. The look in Kurt's eyes says, "Now." Hazel curls up in Kurt's lap, Cole sits next to me in his own chair, and we tell them what we know.

"We found out why Mama has been having headaches. She has a growth in the back of her head called a tumor that needs to come out. We met today with a doctor who wants to do surgery soon," says Kurt.

"I don't like surgeries! I don't want to tell my friends, 'Hi! My mom has a tumor!' " Hazel shouts, then she breaks down in tears and comes over to me, crawling in my lap, and holding me tight. She tries to calm herself down by singing. Hazel sings all the time; she sings while tying her shoes, while making her lunch, and while doing her math homework. Usually, she sings songs that she makes up about whatever she is doing. Once, when she was very young, I taught her to sing "My Favorite Things" from *The Sound of Music* when she was feeling sad. I hadn't heard her sing that song in years. But right now, she pushes out the words between sobs as if she were hanging on to them for dear life. "Raindrops on roses and whiskers on kittens. Brown paper packages tied up with string…"

Cole looks at her and then at me, "Don't worry, Hazel, it's all going to work out. It's all going to be OK." Kurt says, "It won't be easy, but many people have gone through this before and are doing well now. There is still so much we need to find out, and we'll tell you what we learn as soon as we learn it."

"When will you have the surgery?" Cole asks.

"Soon. But no dates yet."

I look at Cole and his face shows only strength. I wonder if he will let himself fall apart.

I don't have to wonder for long. That night, when everyone goes to sleep, Cole finds me in the kitchen and gives me a long, tight hug. He cries into my shoulder. He feels it. And I see now why crying and accepting the tumor as real is important. He says, "I love you, Mama."

"I love you so much, Cole," I say back. If we can face it, we can move forward, together.

7

That weekend, we have plans to go camping with another family in the Rocky Mountains. I tell Kurt and the kids to go without me. I say, "I need to be alone." It is a tough decision. I'm not sure I want to be alone; I want to be in a high meadow, surrounded by wildflowers and the people I love. But the voice inside me whispers, "Go in."

Before Kurt leaves, he looks at me in the eyes and says, "Remember, we're all going to die. The question is, how do you want to *live?*"

I have been sitting on my bed for hours, in the dark, pretending to meditate on that question. My head aches with electric pulses. My throat feels tight, like I am choking. I want to feel calm, but I am agitated.

I pick my journal up off the floor and write, "How do I want to live? It doesn't matter! I am going to die soon. I won't make an impact on the world. I'll never see my kids grow up. My parents will be heartbroken." None of these thoughts feel like fears; they feel like facts.

My mind wanders to the image of the red fox I saw a few days ago while out for a run. The fox was soaked from the rain. Its body looked dark and small with wet fur pressed against its ribs. It ran frantically against traffic on a busy road. The news of this tumor makes me feel like I am running frantically against traffic on a busy road. I can't find anything familiar; I can't reach safe ground.

I have been running my whole life. I have been afraid of standing still and discovering that I am nothing. I believe that if I stop, I'll be nothing. Everyone will run ahead and I will be left behind, alone.

I will die young and without a voice. My children will grow up without a mother.

I am too much in my head and I don't know how to get out of it. It's not a surprise that this tumor is in my skull. I am way out of balance.

I jump up and slam the bedroom door over and over again to drown out Fear's voice. It doesn't work. Then I want the hurt to come out. I kick our metal trash can, hard. Paint flies off the wall where it hits. I kick it again. I want it to break. It only bends and wobbles on the bedroom floor.

I am breathing hard, but I can't get enough air. I feel like someone placed a truck on my chest. There is so much pain. And I can't stop sweating. I reach for my phone to call 911. *I'm having a heart attack!* But before I make the call, I remember what this is; it is not a heart attack; it is an anxiety attack. *Lie down. You've been here before. This too shall pass.*

In a desperate attempt to get the invisible truck off my chest, I take off my clothes and lie on the bed naked. My heart feels like it is exploding out of my body, it is beating so hard and fast. I gently place my hands over my heart and talk to myself. *You're ok. You're alright. You are safe.* Then I try nostril breathing, a trick I learned to quiet my heart. I pinch my right nostril closed, and inhale only through the left. Then I close the left nostril and exhale only through the right. It takes all of my concentration to pinch, breathe, and release. But it is working; I feel slightly calmer.

I feel the coolness of my hands on my bare skin, the curve of my breasts, my sharp elbows and hips, the weight of my skull. I touch the place where spine and skull meet. I don't feel a bump or a bulge. *Where IS this life-threatening tumor?*

My head hurts only slightly; I feel it like a dim pulsing on my fingers. I don't feel like I am choking anymore. I can swallow and breathe. I've stopped sweating. The only thing wrong with me is that Fear is chewing on the neurosurgeon's words and spitting out venomous thoughts. "You didn't make anything of your life. And now it's over."

I don't feel any physical pain. The only things causing me suffering are these negative thoughts.

And then, right there on my bed, among the thousand pillows, something shifts inside me. I feel my mind separate from my thinking. I can see Fear's thoughts as handwriting on a blackboard and my mind as the teacher, reading them. I have sudden and simple clarity that I am not my thoughts. I am the one reading them; that's all. I don't know how I know this; I just do. Before I was afraid of being left alone. Now I see that taking quiet time to myself is the key to finding my inner voice.

I think again, *I will die young and without a voice,* but as the words appear, my mind pulls away and watches them. As I watch, the blackboard seems to absorb the words and they are gone. I feel light, expansive, free. The minute I realize that I don't need to believe all of my thoughts, they vanish. It is sudden and unexpected. It makes me laugh out loud.

Then I hear someone say, *I will come out of this better than before.* And I realize it is my voice. It's not Fear's seductive drawl. It's the quiet-but-spunky voice deep inside me. *Maybe I am not going to die. Maybe I am about to become something new?*

Outside my window, dawn breaks. I see several cedar waxwings, one of my favorite birds, fill the branches of a cherry tree. Their yellow bellies are bright against dark branches. Then they open their wings and take to the air. They move like splashes of sunshine. Now I know why birds can fly. They aren't weighed down by fears of falling.

Years ago, I started writing a memoir, but I never finished it because I was trying to make it perfect. I kept writing and rewriting the first twelve pages. The voice of Fear needled me, "You can't do that! You are not famous or important. Who do you think you are, writing a memoir?" So I put the book away in a box in the basement.

Now, I pull out the dusty, cardboard box. I look at my book. I hear Fear say, "No one wants to read your story." Alone, in the quiet, I listen for my inner voice underneath that one. I hear it. It sounds daring, and it feels like joy. It says, "I don't care who reads it; I want to write it!"

I know how I want to respond to Kurt. I know how I want to live. Alone on my bed, at dawn, I scribble down nine words on my manuscript: *I choose joy over fear, and brave over perfect.*

That night, friends call and invite me out to a movie. I don't want to go, but I say, "Sure." Apparently, listening to my inner voice is harder than I think. The movie that is labeled a comedy is not funny. It is grim; the whole thing is filmed in dark green and brown. It plays the same violin lines of music over and over. People die senseless, graphic deaths. I sit there in pain—not because of my head, but because of the movie. Strangely, I don't think to get up and walk out of the theater. It feels like I have to stay, because that is just what one does. But then I remember how the tumor is growing around my vocal cords, and I repeat my mantra: *I choose joy over fear and brave over perfect.*

When the actors on screen start kicking a dog to death, I lean over to my friend and say, "I'm going to leave now." I crawl awkwardly over her husband's lap and leave the theater.

It's a warm, beautiful night. I go for a walk and watch the sunset behind the mountains. I get a strange sense of exhilaration, so different than the dread I felt in the dark theater. *I walked out.* I would never have done that before; it would have felt weak or just rude. But the idea that I could, and that I did, felt like freedom. Two minutes after I left, a woman who was sitting behind me walked out too. *How many of us were sitting in that theater, waiting for it to get better and not doing anything?*

The movie eventually ends, and my friends meet me outside. I don't know what to expect from them as a response. *Will they ever invite me out again?* They take one look at my smile, and then at the sunset with its bright tangerine clouds, and say, "You didn't miss a thing."

Maybe someday soon I will use my voice to close the gender equity gap, end injustice, and create lasting change in a big way. But for me, walking out of a movie is a brave step toward listening to the voice that's mine and no one else's.

The next day, I wake up and say, "Hello." Kurt says, "Hello?" in a confused, sleepy tone. *Good. My voice still works.* And Kurt is home. They must have returned from camping in the middle of the night. I touch my head, my neck, and my arms. *I'm still alive.* I peek into the room that the kids share. I see their tousled hair and smell their stinky feet. Everyone is where they should be. *Am I safe?* Right now, yes.

I also feel buoyed by the fact that nothing terrible happened when I walked out of the movie last night. As Kurt fries two eggs in a hot skillet this morning, I pause and listen to what I really want to say. Is it the most important thing to tell him that I think his diet is too high in cholesterol? Or is there a feeling that I want to express? I say, "I'm so happy you're home." He smiles and puts his plate down next to mine. "Thank you. I missed you." This is a good way to begin a day. We'll talk later about my experience when I was alone with my thoughts.

8

I keep coming up with reasons why we can't ask for help yet. *Once things calm down. Once we know exactly what we need. Once we have a treatment plan.* But the truth is that asking for help is not in this perfectionist's vocabulary. It's hard to show up as put-together, not needy, and competent if I also have to beg. It's not that I'm against the idea of others lending a hand; I just want to have a plan first.

But today, I notice that all my excuses begin with the word "once." That sounds a lot like procrastination to me. *Once I clean my entire desk, then I'll write.* Beneath procrastination is the familiar voice of Fear. Fear says, "You should wait. Things will get worse and you'll need more help then." "People will feel hassled." "You will have to repay them all."

One night as we walk around the block, Kurt asks, "Really? You think loving somebody is a *hassle?*"

"No, but you have to admit that I can't reciprocate if I can't even take care of myself," I say.

"You're the only one who thinks you have to repay people for loving you," Kurt says.

"So you think we should tell more people than our family?" I ask.

"I think we tell everyone. You never know who might be able to help."

Now I need to find the courage to admit I can't handle this challenge alone. This not only goes against my perfectionist tendencies, it goes against my ancestors.

The words on my grandparents' gravestones might as well say, "Be stoic and don't bother anyone with your troubles." I was born and raised in Toronto, Canada. It's common to hear people in the streets of Toronto saying, "Sorry!" or "Oh! I'm so sorry!" as they apologize for even *potentially* being in someone's path. I'm exaggerating, of course. But underneath this verbal tic of saying "sorry" is a belief that it is better to stay quiet and out of people's way. This self-effacing quality of Canadians is endearing, but can be self-defeating.

Take this strange example of etiquette that I learned as a child. As a guest in someone's home, I remember being told never to ask for food or drink. My mom would say, "If the Queen, or anyone else, offers you a biscuit, turn it down at least twice before accepting. Only on the third offer, say, 'Yes, thank you. That would be lovely.' " Why Mom thought the Queen of England would ever invite us to her palace is another story. Nevertheless, I took the instructions to never appear to need anything to heart. And I was always hungry in people's homes when I moved to the United States because no one in the US offers you something to eat a third time. Americans have this annoying habit of assuming you are genuinely not hungry if you have turned them down twice already.

American culture has its own stigmas against asking for help. Look at some of its favorite heroes: the Lone Ranger, the Man with No Name, and Han Solo. Being brave is synonymous with "going it alone." No wonder it's awkward to ask for help. It puts me squarely in the need-to-be-rescued category when I have always preferred to be the hero.

It therefore takes several sleepless nights before I finally sit down to write an email to everyone in my address book with the subject line, "Serious Curveball: Some Tough News." I explain what we know about the tumor and ask for their positive thoughts. I close my eyes, take a few breaths, and press send.

Once we open the door, loving support comes flooding in. Everyone writes, "How can I help?" It makes me panic a little. I have no idea what to tell them. I don't know what we need. Fear laughs at me and says, "See. It's too soon to ask for help. You need a plan first." But this experience is so new that I don't even know where to begin to make a plan. There is so much to learn and so little time. *Now what do I do with all these people waiting and worrying about me?*

One thing is clear; I have to find a way to update everyone. I look at all the health crisis platforms such as CaringBridge, but I can't get myself to fill in the login page. It makes me cry scrolling through all the stories of sick people. I want to think beyond my current health situation and create a place where people can come for inspiration.

I have been meaning to start a blog for years, but I've never had the guts. With time, I start to see this moment as an opportunity. I have been handed a permission slip to create my own website. It doesn't just have to be about me being sick. I can invite others to write there too. It can be a place of thriving creativity. My panic slowly pivots to excitement.

A young friend connects me with a website creator, Salih Zain, a twenty-year old international student. He is back at home in Iraq for the summer. Despite never having met one another in person, the ten-hour time difference, and navigating the Muslim holiday of Ramadan (which means he fasts for forty days and can only work at night), Salih creates a website for me in less than a week in exchange for a donation toward his education. Then my best friend Natasha's husband, Lorne, creates newsletter templates to send out medical updates, and adds a guestbook space to the website so people can send us messages in one, beautiful space.

Since it is summertime and the kids are out of school, we are struggling to take care of Cole and Hazel while going to all these new doctor visits. Someone suggests we find a "team leader" to organize tasks such as dropping and picking the kids up from camps and bringing us dinner. We decide to try it. I ask Shannon O'Kane, a friend, former colleague, and the most organized person I know, to be my team leader. Each week, we give her a list of logistical issues and she sends out emails to our neighbors, matching the tasks with willing volunteers. The more specific we are with our requests, the better the response. One week we ask for help sorting and copying my medical records, a ride for our daughter to dance class, a ride for our son to a dentist appointment, and for someone to water our lawn. Our friends and neighbors step up generously.

Our children's friends want to contribute, too. It's easy to wonder what they can do, but I am noticing that helping is healing for all of us. Instead of dismissing the kids' requests to help, we give their needs consideration. One week we ask them to draw pictures of me as a funny old lady, vibrant and healthy. Then we ask them to find something natural outside—a rock, a shell, a pine cone—to add to the "altar of goodness" that I created in my bedroom. Next, my dear friend, Sarah Byrden, gives us a great idea. She invites everyone to light a candle every night and speak positive thoughts into the flame. The response is overwhelmingly enthusiastic. I hear stories of friends and their children in Senegal and Bolivia, Nepal and the Netherlands, lighting candles each night. And I can feel it working. I feel less heavy, full of light.

⁂

Once I accept that the world is not going to spin off its axis if I ask for help, I create a series of silly, thirty-second videos to entertain people. It is important to me to counter their feelings of fear and helplessness. I convince my dear friend Teresa to make the videos with her old iPhone. We do all of them in one or two takes, not trying to perfect them, just knocking them out, cracking ourselves up.

The videos include a reprise of the song "I Will Survive" done with Kurt on the guitar, and "Where is the Love?" done karaoke-style, in

Teresa's car. In another video, I dress up as Julie Andrews in *The Sound of Music* and run over a hill singing "I have confidence!" You can hear Teresa laughing in that one. In a third video, I am talking to the tumor. "When you feel the surgeon's hands on you, you need to let go completely." My thinking is that if others see me talk to the tumor, maybe they'll be brave enough to talk to it as well. The tumor might actually listen to a chorus of voices and leave quietly, forever.

Making these low-quality, slapstick movies is how my voice first tests the waters before asking for financial help. Because of how rare my condition is, and the complex nature of the required surgeries, we will likely need to go out of state, and definitely outside of our insurance company's network, to get experienced care. We have no idea how much our insurance company will cover of our incurred costs, and if I will ever be able to work again.

But I can't bring myself to ask for money. I put ads on Craigslist to sell our car, my bike, and my jewelry, without telling Kurt. A nice man comes to look at the car, and asks me why I am selling it. When I tell him, he says, "How will you go to doctors' appointments? How will your kids get to school?" He hands me back the keys. He has a point. Maybe there is another way.

I think about our children and how they might need support in the future. That makes it easier for me to say yes to a fundraising campaign. This requires one more video message. The procrastination begins again. *Once I have a surgery date, I'll start a campaign. Once we know what everything will cost, I'll make the video.* One day, my friend Catherine wraps her arm around my shoulders and firmly walks me outside. She gives me a pep talk and then films me in our backyard, telling my story. I sit on an overturned wooden crate and she stands above me. The message is meant to be serious, but because she is so tall, the video is slightly humorous; I am craning to look all the way up at her.

I have to say some of the most difficult words I have ever spoken, and I have to say them into a camera. "I want to be out there, giving to the world instead of asking you for help, but I need your help. In order to get through this, we need your positive visualizations and your financial support."

My voice shakes. I'm going to cry. But I don't want to do a second take. I perk up again at the end when I take the time to thank everyone. My voice is steady when I say, "I want you to know that your love and prayers are already working. I now have the strength to see this as an opportunity to shake off my fear and step into my full power, which is exactly what the world needs all of us to do."

These words are meant to start a fundraising drive that my friends Natasha, Alli, and Teza call "Love & Courage." Only I won't allow my friends to release the video or announce the campaign. "Once things calm down, we can do it," I tell them. Old habits die hard. I stall. I think, *Not now. Not yet.*

Not knowing my future makes me anxious. To calm my anxiety, I hold tightly to anything that gives me a feeling of control. Today, it is pickles.

I am standing in a crowded supermarket aisle, shopping with Kurt for my brother's family barbecue.

"My family doesn't like those kinds of pickles. My family prefers dills," I say to Kurt, taking the pickles he has chosen out of the cart, and putting them back on the shelf.

"Really? Well, who exactly is included in your family? Am *I* included in your family? Because if so, I prefer bread and butter pickles," Kurt responds, as he places the jar of thinly sliced pickles back in the cart. As we wrestle the jar out of each other's hands, I break down. I am laughing, then crying, in the middle of the narrow aisle. A woman tries to move past me to continue her shopping, but quickly realizes it is no use. I'm buckled over with grief and I can't stand up. She gives me a look of sympathy, then does a twelve-point turn with her cart to find another way out.

A friend encourages me to go see a therapist. On my first visit, I tell the therapist that I've heard that married couples don't always weather a medical crisis well. I confess that I am worried that the fight with Kurt means our relationship is in trouble. Michael, the therapist, listens patiently, then smiles.

"You are worried that the fight you had with Kurt over pickles might crumble everything? I doubt it. Remember, the world is spinning in an expanding universe and you are not in control. Let go."

He is blunt. And, he is right. Every time my mind fights for control of our situation, the more suffering I feel. I have to receive this tumor as reality. My challenge is not to fix the fights with Kurt, work harder, or be stronger. My challenge is to let go.

"But isn't letting go preparing for death?" I ask Michael.

"What's wrong with that?" he asks in return.

"It feels like I'm giving up," I confess.

"Maybe it's the opposite. By facing death, you're embracing life fully."

I am not convinced. But I am curious when he tells me about a local woman who guides people through death meditations. He scribbles her phone number on a piece of paper like a prescription and hands it to me. I call and make an appointment.

Having never met her, I imagine that a woman who leads death meditations will be wearing a flowing robe, a heavy turquoise beaded necklace, and a belt of bones that rattles as she walks.

When she opens the door to her home, I am surprised that she looks like me: a white, middle-aged, skinny chick in jeans. She invites me into her office in the basement of her home that doubles as a guest room. She sits on a chair while I sit on the bed on a soft brown blanket with the image of a wolf woven into it. It's the kind of blanket you might buy at a rest stop in Arizona from a man in an AC/DC t-shirt. I am nervous about this experience, but I am also intrigued.

She tells me that she was once very sick with a mysterious digestive disease that threatened her life. This close call led her to examine her own relationship with death as well as life. She began a path of healing through meditation and deep emotional work around death and dying. Now she guides others through the process.

I sit comfortably on the wolf blanket with my eyes open. Then my guide asks me to look out at the room using only my peripheral vision, while simultaneously feeling any sensations on the top of my head and the bottoms of my feet.

"Looking and noticing this way will help you expand. Spaciousness and curiosity are the secret keys to letting go," she says matter-of-factly. Then she has me close my eyes.

"Think about death," she directs me gently.

I picture a dark tunnel or a hole. I imagine falling. Then I see my children, confused, and spinning into darkness without their mother. I try to feel the sensations at the top of my head, but I'm starting to panic a little. I can't feel my feet at all. After what feels like a long time, she says, "Now imagine a time when you felt held and safe. Describe it to me."

"After the diagnosis, when my husband said he would switch places with me if he could. I felt completely held," I say, feeling the warmth of the memory.

"Keep your eyes closed and soak in that feeling," she instructs. After several minutes, she asks, "How do you feel?"

"I feel safe. I feel loved, strong, and radiant," I answer honestly.

"Did someone do something to make you feel that way just now?"

"No. I'm not sure what you mean," I say, my eyes still closed.

"Without anyone's help, you were able to feel loved, strong, radiant. Death can feel that comfortable too."

"But what about how it feels to the people who are still alive?"

"They'll feel it if you feel it. You can pass on that feeling of safety, love, and strength to your kids by giving them love now and having them sense how relaxed you are about whatever happens."

"But wait. I felt something else too."

"Tell me about it."

"I felt like I was splitting in two, like there was this zipper between two parts of me, one that was sitting down calmly, feeling safe and strong, and another that was restless and shouting scary things at me."

"There is your essential self, your soul, and there is your scared self that fights change and wants control. The scared self is afraid of losing its power, so it will shout 17,000 fear-filled thoughts a minute at you. No matter what that scared self is saying, your essential self is always there, strong and calm."

"But does the splitting mean I am dying?"

"I think you're transforming; the scared self is dying because it doesn't serve you anymore. Meanwhile, the essential self is coming alive more than ever."

We are wading in deep waters on the edge of my comfort zone. It's a lot to take in. But I can absorb most of what she is saying. I understand that my desire to control everything isn't working anymore to make me feel safe. The only thing that works is to accept that I have a tumor and accept that my future is uncertain. *I can't do that. I don't want this tumor. It makes me angry.* I have to accept my feelings, too. I know that I *prefer* to live in this body, on this green earth, as a mother to my children. But I may not get what I prefer.

I let go of control in one small way. On my way home, my childhood friend Teza calls.

"Are you ready to let us fundraise for you?" she asks. If I say yes, the tumor is real. There is no going back to my life before the diagnosis. *Can I accept that?*

I remember my experience just moments before. *They'll feel it if you feel it.*

"Yes, I'm ready," I tell Teza.

9

We decide to call it "*the* tumor" instead of "*my* tumor," in case it gets the wrong message and thinks it is welcome to stay in my body. My brother and the kids also call it "the Macarena" after that wedding-dance song that often gets stuck in your head against all wishes. If I knew the tumor's scientific name, I know what I would do. I'd type it into Google and obsessively read everything there is about it.

Kurt already tried. He searched every kind of skull-base tumor and found pages and pages of frightening statistics, average life spans, and generalized information, non-specific to my case. But no one knows what kind of tumor it is; the doctors won't even know until *after* the surgeries. I decide to stay offline. Kurt does research for both of us, and shares with me only what's needed, relevant, and positive.

My drive to load up on information comes from a desire to intelligently prepare for what lies ahead. It's how I have survived in the past. But now it could be marching me down the wrong path. It gives me a false sense of control. The consequences of rushing toward answers that will always be incomplete is that I don't actually face my feelings. Now I see that I'm looking for a way out through information. There is no way out of my new reality. Something tells me that I need to look for a way in. I want to learn to face pain, discomfort, anger, and fear.

In the meantime, we spend our days sending the images of my skull to surgeons that Kurt finds online. Then we wait for them to call us back. I remember one conference call with a team of superstar neurosurgeons in Los Angeles. Kurt puts them on speakerphone as we sit at the kitchen table. We take turns asking our short list of questions.

"How many surgeries have you performed in your career?" Kurt asks.

"Oh, upwards of five thousand," the principal neurosurgeon answers.

"How many surgeries with this set of risks have you done before?"
I ask.

"Uh, well. No one can say they've done a lot like this," the
surgeon answers.

"What can we expect when looking around for the right person to
operate?" Kurt asks.

"If someone tells you that they've done more than two dozen surgeries
like this, don't believe them," the neurosurgeon cautions us. I stand
up from the table and walk toward the window. It hits me just how
difficult my situation is and how we might not find someone to help.
Kurt thanks the surgeons and hangs up the phone. We both take some
deep breaths. We inhale the reality and exhale helplessness.

Then I remember that I actually know a neurosurgeon. I call Dr.
Moustapha Abou-Samra. He immigrated to the US from Syria, and
is the father of two of my former students. I haven't spoken to him
in twenty years. He returns my call and seems genuinely happy to be
reconnected. He asks me to send the MRI scans. In a few days, he calls
me back.

"You didn't tell me how serious this is!" He says, full of heart.

"I was hoping you would tell me that it's no big deal," I say.

"I want to help you more than anything, but this is very complex. You
need to call the finest skull-based tumor specialists. Here are a few
names. I went to medical school in Syria with one of the very best. His
name is Dr. Ossama Al-Mefty. He's in Boston."

"You know what I think when I see a Muslim man in the airport?" Kurt asks me as we wait in the security line at the airport. The kids are staying with friends while we travel to Boston.

"What?" I look around nervously, wondering where this might be going.

"Neurosurgeon," Kurt says, and smiles.

We are on our way to meet with Dr. Al-Mefty, the world's leading expert on skull-base tumors. He immigrated from a predominately Muslim country. At Brigham and Women's Hospital in Boston, his waiting room is packed with people: children with their worried parents, young men in business suits, older men in ball caps with the words "US VET" embroidered in all-capital letters.

The TVs in the waiting room are turned up, loud, broadcasting the Republican National Convention. I can't escape the nominee's voice, shouting, "We need to build a wall and make America safe again!" I open my journal to write down what I see and feel. I am sensitive to the word "safe." It's attractive. Who doesn't want to feel safe? Who doesn't want to protect their family from harm? We can't block out risk or insulate ourselves from danger. We can only respond.

Sitting in this hospital, it is clear to me that the harm does not come from immigrants. They actually seem to be the ones running this hospital, and caring for everyone. Earlier, I heard the nominee say, "We need a total and complete shutdown of Muslims entering the United States."

Are these the same Muslims known for their expertise in solving complex neurosurgical problems? And the ones who clean bed pans and do the hospital laundry? The ones who spend every waking minute saving the lives of Americans of all faiths and ethnicities?

According to this presidential candidate, our country's problems are clearly the fault of these "nasty, no-good immigrants."

Then, a Haitian nurse calls us into an examining room. Dr. Al-Mefty meets us there. It is after six o'clock at night. He is giving up dinner with his family to help Kurt and me understand the risks involved with operating on the tumor. He articulates a more aggressive approach that any other surgeon we've spoken to, one that involves going after every piece of the tumor, despite the risks.

At the end of the visit, Kurt and I decide quietly to ask Dr. Al-Mefty to perform my surgeries. We choose him because of his unparalleled skill and experience, not to mention his complete devotion to his patients, regardless of their background. *But hey, shut those borders down! We don't need any more smart, dedicated people in this country!*

I type up my thoughts about this experience, then hit "publish blog" before I have time to second-guess my writing. This post is especially vulnerable for me because it is political. The next thing that happens surprises me. I receive an email from a friend in New York. Her husband is an actor who works on the show *Homeland*.

"I hope it's OK that I talked to the producers of *Homeland* about your recent post. They are looking for ways to expand their portrayal of Muslims on the show. Now they are considering adding a neurosurgeon character." I am stunned, and happy. My little voice might make an impact.

It doesn't make sense to find my voice now, in hospital waiting rooms and airports. But then again, falling in love never makes sense. And it feels like I am falling in love with writing again. Writing feels healing. Writing feels like being home.

We call Dr. Al-Mefty back to say that we'd be honored if he would perform the craniotomies. He responds that the surgeries will take approximately thirty-six hours, over three consecutive days. He admits that his schedule is full, but that he will make time for me. We are grateful, and nervous. *Will he be able to see me in time?*

10

Kurt and I are standing in our kitchen, after the kids have fallen asleep. We're cleaning up after dinner when the phone rings. It's Dr. Al-Mefty, calling us himself.

"The surgery will take two days. I can operate in one month, on August first and second. After that, my next six months are very busy. And in your case, I don't think you should wait that long," he says.

"Wonderful!" Kurt says, grateful that the surgery can happen soon. I shake my head "no" in silence and take a step back from the phone. Kurt looks at me with a worried expression.

"Thank you. We'll get back to you right away about those dates," says Kurt. He ends the call and turns to me.

"Have you changed your mind? Do you not want to go through with the surgeries?" Kurt asks.

"No. I do. But if I die, does it have to be on Cole's birthday?"

"Oh, hon. Can you imagine a different outcome? One that has our son celebrating his birthday and the successful removal of the tumor? Or one where Cole is fine, regardless of the outcome?"

"I don't know."

I go for a walk alone. The moon looks ragged behind dark clouds. At first, the streetlights help me to see where I am going, but then I head up hill, off the main street. It is so dark I can't tell what is ahead of me, or behind.

In a dark time, the eye begins to see.

So begins a poem by Theodore Roethke. My high school students and I used to sit and read the lines of this poem out loud together. I remember doing this on the anniversary of 9/11. And again when one of my students was paralyzed in a bike accident, and again when a faculty member's brother died.

I know the purity of pure despair

My shadow pinned against a sweating wall—

In this dark time, I see finally that I am afraid. I see that I have been listening to the news and mourning the end of the world. Horrible shootings. Senseless, irreparable violence. Politicians screaming offensive remarks, clouding the air with hatred. A people divided and afraid. I see, too, that I am already grieving my own death. Fear sits on my shoulder and whispers in my ear, "Cole's thirteenth birthday will be the day his mom died."

I want to return to childhood, when things seemed simpler and happier. I don't want to make decisions that involve pain. I don't want a government that doesn't believe in climate change or telling the truth. I don't want to have these operations. I don't want to die. And I really don't want to die on my son's birthday.

Even though I am walking on a smooth sidewalk as an adult, I feel like a child, I imagine that I am on a narrow path through the forest at night, without a flashlight. It takes all of my senses to move forward. I have to listen, feel, and taste my next step. *Do I know for sure that I am going to die?* No. *Do I know for sure that these politicians are going to burn the world to ashes?* No. It's been dark before. It will be dark again. We can still move forward in the dark.

I slowly let my eyes adjust. And now I see a deer, feeding on my neighbor's lawn. She lifts her head to look at me.

As I approach, she makes three high bounds away from me. Then she stops, and stands still. Kurt has a PhD in wildlife biology. I remember him telling me that a doe, when it senses the danger of a mountain lion approaching, leaps away, but for no more than fifteen minutes. Then she listens, and slowly relaxes. She calmly licks the dew from the grass. She recovers fully so that if the lion approaches again, she will be able to escape.

But lately, I am living in Fear's grasp all the time. I feel threatened, unsafe, and out of control. My body can't tell that there isn't a lion. The result is that I am trying to live, parent, and make decisions from the core of a nervous system that is only designed to help me for fifteen minutes at a time, to immediately escape danger.

The deer watches me, unafraid. I walk past, moving easily now, somehow able to see the path in the dark. *Is it really true that the world and I can't survive this dark time?*

I remember feeling overwhelmed by the unknowns when I was pregnant and about to give birth to Cole. I wanted my doctor to reassure me that nothing terrible would happen in delivery. I wanted the baby to be healthy and perfect. At thirty-eight weeks pregnant, I sat in my doctor's office and said, "I feel overwhelmed by all of the things that could go wrong with this baby."

My doctor, a wise woman, suggested, "Why don't you spend more time imagining how things could go right?"

I climb out of my fear.

These times are uncertain, but are not *all* times uncertain? *How then should I live?*

In these dark times, I see that there is no recipe for safety. There is no way to predict the light or wash away the darkness. If I let them operate on my son's birthday, I may die on the table. If I put off the surgeries, I may die waiting.

I can spend my time stuck in fear, fury, and fed-up-ness. Or I can step through the darkness. He is strong. I am strong. Twenty-four of the thirty-six hours of surgery on my skull, brain, and spine will take place on Cole's thirteenth birthday. I raise my thoughts from *I will die* to *I will come out of this more alive than before.*

With my students, we used to linger on the confusing last line of Roethke's poem, trying to make sense of it.

And one is One, free in the tearing wind.

Right now, I see the lowercase, singular "one" as me sitting in the dark, facing my personal fears. And I see the capitalized "One" as all of us, together. We are tiny. We are massive.

It's about time I see myself as massive, and my thoughts as influential. In these uncertain times, I remember I am not alone. The way forward for me to heal is through the universal. We are all in pain. Someone loses his job, a child gets sick, a parent dies, a fire burns the family home, and we struggle to get up in the morning because we think we are not worthy. No one is immune from suffering. Maybe in the process of being in the dark together, we heal and set each other free.

I walk back to the house, my eyes fully adjusted now. I open the door and find some scrap paper. I am determined to write Cole a letter for Kurt to give him on his birthday. I sit down at our kitchen table and write Cole until late into the night. I want to write Hazel too, but I'm exhausted. I will write her, just not tonight. Then I crawl in bed, next to Kurt.

"What do you want to tell Dr. Al-Mefty?" he asks me, groggily.

"Those dates are fine, thank you," I say with surprising confidence.

"Are you sure?" Kurt rolls over to look at me in the eyes.

"Yes."

⁓⁘⁓

Dear Cole,

When you were three years old, we went for a walk along the muddy banks of the Connecticut River in Lyme, New Hampshire. It was raining and we watched the swallows feed off the recently-hatched bugs on the surface of the water. You identified raccoon tracks in the mud and said, "They look like tiny hands, Mama." This memory makes me so indescribably happy.

And now you are turning thirteen and we still we walk together. Well, I walk, and you skateboard. We head up the hill to see the view of the Rocky Mountains and just how much sky there is to see in Colorado. Then I hold my breath while you turn away and ride down the steep section of Alpine Avenue. You carve wide turns, picking up speed, and arch your back to balance as you lean into the hill and read the ground with your body.

I have always loved walking with you and paying attention to the world as we go. Some of your first words were "Mama in mud." Your first sentence was, "Toad peed on Mama." These were your very first stories, born in the adventures of us heading outside, exploring, with no idea where we would end up. We're kind of on a walk now as we face the unknowns of my surgeries and the unknowns of your teenage years.

When I try to remember my teenage self, I recall the way I carved bright blue eyeliner into my bottom eyelid to try to fit in with others, and I wore a black leather jacket to stand out. It was a bewildering time, full of the pushes and pulls of wanting to blend in and wanting to be different.

I wish someone had said to me: Instead of fitting in, figure out where you belong. For that you need to learn to try less hard. Pay attention to what you like and what you don't like, and you will feel your way into belonging.

These are the years when you practice making and keeping friends. Practice is the key word here. Make friends with lots of different kinds of people—girls, too. It takes more effort, but it's worth it. People who are different from you teach you the most. There isn't a shortcut to figuring out relationships; you have to go through it all. One minute you'll feel like you belong; the next, rejected; the next, betrayed; the next, accepted. It's all very confusing. Remember, when you feel left out, it's not because your friends got together and planned to ignore you, but rather because they're a bunch of human beings swimming around in their own emotional soup. You're still just dumb kids learning and growing. As our dear friend Sue Kruse says, "You are a work in progress."

As a work in progress, be kind to yourself. I wasted too much energy on trying to make everyone happy, and when that didn't work out, I spent too much time being hard on myself. It's important not to give in to thoughts about not being good enough, because you cannot be kind to others if you are not kind to yourself. It's like trying to dance with a partner without moving your feet.

Your Papa told me once that he never knew what he wanted to do as a teenager. "My friends and I didn't do anything but hang out because we didn't want something interesting to happen and miss it. So we just sat around in Vinay Kwatro's basement, waiting for something to happen, and nothing ever did."

Don't wait too long. Create the life you want to live. When the end comes, all that fear of fitting in and all the worry and waiting will be for nothing. I have had a magnificent life, but I put off my desire to write and make my writing public because I was afraid of these two unanswerable questions: *How will I make money?* And: *Who will care about what I have to say?* The answers don't matter anymore. I am motivated to write because I will regret it if I don't, period.

I won't always be able to walk with you through dark times. This is the pain of parenting. But I believe that everything you need to thrive is within you. We are capable of far more than we think.

When dark times come, remember: joy is a much more powerful force than fear. But you have to be fierce to stop listening to other voices, and to start listening to your own. Underneath your fear is joy. Let joy lead and you will walk through anything with courage and curiosity.

The only other thing I want to tell you right now is that none of what is happening to me is your responsibility. And what I mean is that you may feel the need to be strong for Hazel or for Papa. Or you may feel really sad or angry. You may feel nothing at all. I have felt all of these ways, sometimes in the space of five minutes. But everyone is going to respond differently and that is not just normal, it is necessary. Be patient with yourself. There is nothing you can do to change what is and I believe there is a deeper, loving intelligence at play that will make sure that all will be well.

I am not afraid right now. I feel so loved and held. And I feel so connected to you, so in love and grateful for our amazing family. Thank you for making me laugh all the time; your quick wit is one of your many gifts. Please give of your humor generously because you can change a mood from dark to light in a heartbeat.

You and I have many more walks together and I can't wait to explore the world with you. Our connection is not one that lives only in the physical world; it is much wider and deeper than that.

Happy Birthday, Cole. I love you, unconditionally. Go into the world knowing that and watch the way the world responds back with love.

Love,
Mama

11

What happens next takes my breath away. Once we announce the surgery dates and I allow the fundraising campaign to launch, I get a crash course in learning to receive. People give. They give generously. Many others write to us and say, "I don't have any extra money right now, but each day I picture you healthy and laughing in the sunshine." It all helps. We reach our goal quickly. We immediately send out a note saying, "Thank you. We did it! Put your wallets away!" Yet they keep on giving.

Neighbors bring us groceries, do our laundry, bake us bread, mow our lawn, even weatherize our porch. Children send us drawings and homemade cupcakes. Colleagues create a regular meeting time for positive visualizations. Kurt and I cry a lot these days, out of gratitude.

Our friends are teaching me that "to receive" is an active verb. It's always felt submissive to me; I've never wanted to sit back and take what comes to me. But I am learning that receiving is not passive; it is an action. It is the necessary half of an exchange that strengthens relationships.

If you knew that you were loved, how would you act? I've been thinking about that question lately. It's a twist on the old prompt, What would you do if money were no object? I don't think we know how much we matter to others. I certainly had no idea. I've spent my life trying to prove that I am worthy of love. If I knew that I was already loved, I would hustle less. I would stop trying to be everything to everyone. I would take more risks. Speak up more. Dance in public. Worry less. Be bold more often.

What if our aversion to asking for help is holding us back from experiencing what we most need: to be loved unconditionally? Most people don't experience community until it is too late, at their funeral. I feel lucky to feel the love now.

A friend sends me a note with a single question, What gifts help? I write her back a list of the unexpected kindnesses that keep me focused on joy instead of fear.

- Emails or texts with no questions. It's too tiring to respond to questions. One friend sends me texts regularly with no words, only pictures of different flowers in her garden. Another sends me a weird emoji often, just to let me know she is thinking of me.

- Handmade art (with a small "a") and handwritten letters. One friend writes me a card every day with a poem. A group of colleagues made me prayer flags, each writing a note on a scrap piece of fabric and tying them together.

- Gift cards to grocery stores, restaurants, and cleaning services.

- Delivered meals or fresh fruit (every *other* day…not enough fridge space for every day).

- Names of bodyworkers, healers, etc.

- Silly video messages. I like the ones where the kids get involved and tell me a joke or show off their latest soccer/skateboard/ piano trick.

- Pajamas, slippers, bathrobe, socks, or a zippered sweatshirt for cold hospital rooms.

- Books. (I like ones about overcoming illness and alternative treatments, but that's just me.)

- Music playlists or movie suggestions (funny and light; or adventurous, daring, and inspiring).

- Care packages. A colleague just helped me to put together care packages for the kids. I wrote cards in advance, then she collected fun games and craft projects. She plans to mail them as if they are from me when I go to the hospital.

It's so simple, really. The gifts that help are not so much things as they are gestures that show me that I don't have to do this alone. With each kind word, I am being carried through this.

For a week, I sleep no more than four hours a night. Then one night I wake up because of the pounding headache at the base of my skull and I spin in thoughts, wondering if I am going to die, or worse, be horribly debilitated. Anyway, I should be exhausted. I should be dragging my body around like a bag of potatoes, but instead I feel energized. It must be from all this support flooding in from everywhere. I feel lifted and light.

Everyone deserves to feel this outpouring of love. *Why do we hold back?* I have said "I love you" more in the past few weeks than I have all year. I have heard it said back to me so often that it feels like "I love you" is my first name and "Susie" is my last name.

What Kurt and I really don't expect is the number of people who thank *us*. We don't understand. They keep saying, "Thank you for bringing us together as a community around something meaningful." We learn this lesson: When you invite someone to help you, you strengthen their sense of connectedness as well as your own.

One night, a former student delivers a hand-bound book full of letters from other former students, expressing their gratitude.

I started teaching high school at twenty-one years old. I looked and sounded more like the students than the faculty. I spent a lot of energy trying to show up as strong, knowledgeable, and grown-up. I was embarrassed by my flaws and tendencies to be silly and I thought I had hidden these traits from my students. In their letters, I see that I wasn't hiding anything.

> *"I will never forget the moment I was stressed about something and you cut short our meeting to jump in a leaf pile. I had never jumped in one before and never thought it was appropriate to, until then."*

All those years, I didn't feel smart enough or literary enough or organized enough to be anyone's teacher.

> *"Let your jaw slacken. Let your pen run. The world will be better for it." You wrote these words to me on a post-it note. I've tried to live by these words ever since."*

> *"The last time we spoke, I had just received the news that I had been rejected from almost all of the colleges I had applied to and was left with only two choices, both of which I was less than enthusiastic about. You reminded me that there were more options than the two envelopes in front of me, and that whatever path I took, I would make it my own."*

The students' letters don't thank me for the few perfect classes that I practically killed myself to teach. They write about the imperfect times when I fell out of a tree teaching Robert Frost's poem, "Birches" or cried while reading Mary Oliver out loud. When I showed up as me, I gave them permission to be fully them.

> *"You taught me that I can be myself. I have taken up Olympic weightlifting. I struggle with the thought that a woman shouldn't be involved in something so manly. But your writing reminds me that I don't need to be everyone else's idea of perfect; I can be happy doing what I love. There's a point when you're at the bottom of a lift, when the weight seems heaviest. It's called "the hole." When you're in the hole, it seems impossible to stand up. My thought when I am in the hole is, "If I can stand up, I will be stronger for it." I imagine the weight you are feeling*

seems immeasurably heavy, like you are in the hole. But I know you will
stand up."

The letters floor me. I open the book, read a page, and then close it
again because I am crying too hard. I wasted so many days comparing
myself to teachers I knew or had. I was convinced I would never
be a great teacher, because I measured myself against others with
more experience, more degrees, or more charisma. I beat myself
up constantly for not having the right personality or all the right
answers. I wanted to be someone else, someone who *knew* how to be a
master teacher.

But the students in these letters are saying, "We like *you*, as you." I
wanted to be perfect. But these letters show me that if I had waited
until I was perfect, I would have missed getting to know these amazing
individuals, and missed my chance to make a positive imprint on
their lives.

I don't believe that kind of appreciation is reserved for teachers,
leaders, or special people. It is available for everyone; it's just tough to
figure out how to invite it into our lives.

Humans want to love, to give, and to feel connected. It's our most
natural state. My family, friends, and students are teaching me this.

Now I see how I want to behave. Bold. Loving. True. Reading the
letters from my students, I am inspired. I will use my voice to thank
the people who have guided me, without waiting any longer. I begin
by calling my parents. Then I call mentors and friends. *Why do we
wait so long to tell people how important they have been to us?* I don't want to
wait anymore.

I know now that when I have the opportunity to give, I will give.
And when I have an opportunity to receive, I will receive. I want to
embrace fully both sides of the gift.

12

In two days, we fly to Boston. I'm packing letters for my family in case I don't survive. I'm also packing slippers to wear after surgery when I live. I am preparing to die. I am also preparing to live. And now I'm wondering about life after death.

The first time I remember thinking about life after death is in the fall of 1990. I am a second-year student at Middlebury College, a small liberal arts college in Vermont. My advisor is Chaplain Walsh, a brilliant, kind man. He invites me to his office one Friday and asks me to forego my plans to leave campus that weekend.

"I want to ask a favor of you," he says with a serious tone in his voice. I adore Chaplain Walsh and I will do anything for him, but I don't want to say yes because I am really excited to get off campus for a couple of days.

"There is a conference at the college this weekend. I need you to give a tour to a special guest named Dolly," He says clearly, and definitively. I don't know how to say no to him, so I say yes and let go of my plan of leaving for the weekend.

"How will I know how to find Dolly?" I ask.

"Be at the chapel at 10 a.m."

With bedhead and bleary eyes after a full night of college-style partying, I arrive at the meeting spot the next morning. The chapel sits at the top of a long, sloping hill. There is a single paved path that cuts through the grass to the chapel steps. It is a foggy, damp morning in Vermont. I imagine that Dolly might be blonde, like Dolly Parton, but I don't see anyone who looks like that on the path. All I see is a group of men in robes with shaved heads, making their way toward me. Monks! I think. What are they doing here?

"Good morning," I say. "Are you lost?"

They respond by bowing before me, smiling and nodding. I bow awkwardly back.

"I am Susie. A student. I'm waiting for someone named Dolly."

"Ah! Good. This is Dolly." The cloud of saffron-and-wine robes part and a short, older man in glasses steps forward. He gives me a wide smile that makes his cheeks round like apples. Then he claps his hands together at his chest and bows before me. I don't know who this man is, but I see and feel intense white light wrapped all around him, and now me. I instinctively bow in response. He touches my head with his.

"This is his High Holiness the 14th Dalai Lama of Tibet," says one of the young monks. "Can you help us find the dining room?"

I'm too embarrassed to admit that I have no idea what he just said or who this man is. I know nothing about Tibet. I am a non-religious student who just does what her advisor tells her to do. But I do know where the dining hall is. I lead the posse across the street and into Proctor Hall. It takes a conversation with a wiser student to figure out that I am guiding the Nobel Peace Prize winner and the spiritual leader of Tibet, the Dalai Lama, to the salad bar.

Chaplain Walsh walks over and bows deeply in front of the Dalai Lama, then gives me a hug.

"Why didn't you tell me who I was meeting?" I scold Chaplain Walsh in a whisper.

"It's more fun this way," He winks at me.

The Dalai Lama loves to eat, I discover. When I ask his Holiness if he would like stir-fry or pasta, the Dalai Lama nods twice. His translator says, "Both, please." I show my charge where the bread is and he loads several bagels and cheeses on his plate. Then he fills a bowl with fried potatoes, another bowl with soup, and another with nuts. His little plastic tray is overflowing, so I offer to carry his juice and tea for him on my tray. We sit down at a round table and he motions for me to pass him something. I offer him his juice, then his tea, but he wants my dinner roll!

"What are you studying?" He asks me, with the help of his translator. By now, there are dozens of students and professors gathering around, bowing, and bringing up chairs to sit with us. The Dalai Lama smiles and welcomes each person warmly. Then he looks back at me and waits for my answer.

"Poetry," I say quickly.

"Good for the mind. Does it make you happy?"

"Yes. But others study more important things like international economics," I say, motioning to the people in the growing crowd.

"Do not compare yourself to others. You don't know their journey. Maybe you will help people with poetry," his translator says to me after the Dalai Lama speaks for a minute. Then he laughs.

His Holiness laughs continuously, as though he shares an inside joke with life. He also has a thing for wristwatches. I always assumed that leaders were reserved and serious, especially spiritual ones. But here is the Dalai Lama playing with my watch like a toddler, laughing heartily, and eating like a ravenous retiree at a free all-you-can-eat buffet.

I want to know more about this "Dolly" person who walks in a force field of light. I end up spending the whole weekend serving the Dalai

Lama and his entourage, long after my official duties are over. The conference the college is hosting is on the relationship between religion and the environment, and much to my embarrassment, the biggest attraction is my charge, the Dalai Lama. As I learn about his life in exile from the country he loves, I want to understand what makes a man who has suffered so much capable of such deep kindness.

The Dalai Lama gives several talks. He gets the most animated when he speaks about integrating diverse religions. He says, "It is a human's responsibility to serve, to help others. It is not enough to care for those within one religion. We need to unite all religions and care for others and the earth we share."

What comes to me now are his thoughts on death. I don't remember exactly what he said, but I recall him expressing something like, "The worst thing that can happen is not that you may die. You will die. The worst thing is to die without knowing yourself."

"Why do we avoid the subject of death in our culture?" I ask Chaplain Walsh afterwards.

"If we don't talk about it, we don't have to die," He says with a straight face. Then breaks into a laugh.

I am changed by the end of the weekend. I am fascinated by the connection between life, death, and reincarnation. I remember how I felt a strong light around the Dalai Lama before I knew anything about him, and I remember how much he laughed. I am determined to know more about the light that can shine out of one life.

Six years later, I am on a tiny plane to Lhasa, the capital city of Tibet. I make a deal with a cross-cultural education organization to pay me to chaperone a group of students to Nepal and Tibet. It's the same organization I will later direct.

Just a few days into our trip in Tibet, a young monk named Norbu latches on to us as our guide. He announces joyfully that we are just in time for a sky burial, a Tibetan funeral ceremony. We are visiting Drigung Thil, a mountaintop monastery that was looted and destroyed in 1959 by the Chinese government. When we arrive in 1996, the monks are slowly rebuilding it, by hand.

Two monks carry the body of an old woman on a makeshift stretcher to the stone platform at the center of the meadow. The body is wrapped carefully in white silk ceremonial scarves called *katas*. They lie her down among stones and ribbons of smoke ascending from burning incense. A large group of monks from the monastery sit cross-legged in the distance, chanting.

We stand about fifty feet away. I notice their sharp knives, the white bones, the slender cuts of flesh, and how little blood there is. Suddenly, half of the monks rise. But wait. They are not men; they are giant vultures sitting patiently among the monks. I watch as the vultures spread their wings, extend their long, turkey-like necks, and pounce on the stone platform. They clean the body by separating flesh from bone. The whole thing is over in a couple of minutes. Only bones remain. I grew up thinking of death as final, and as tragic. This feels less like a ritual to mark the end of a life and more of a ceremony to honor her transition from living to dying to living again.

I see the calm excitement on Norbu's face. I watch the vultures beat their powerful wings and launch into the sky. They soar high above us until they are only dots, like bits of ash floating above a fire. It seems generous and natural to give your body to the animals, rather than let it sit wastefully in a coffin or use up a cord of firewood to cremate it. I watch the birds glide overhead against a clear, blue sky and hear only the sound of the wind combing feathers. I wonder, *What's it like to be caught in the throat of a vulture? What does it feel like to fly?*

If death is dark and mysterious, it is also full of wings and light. We transform from human to bird to sky. *What is so frightening about that?*

⁂

Twenty years later, I wake in my home in Colorado with a single thought, "I want a ceremony." I want to mark this moment in my life as a transition, not an ending. For that, I need help. I feel suddenly that I am going to come out of this alive, but not the same. Maybe I'll even have wings.

Nine women gather in my backyard, really just a strip of dead grass, and we sit on blankets and towels in a circle. I ask my friend Genny to lead us in some kind of blessing. She has never led a ceremony like this before, but she says yes anyway. That's what I love about my friends.

I ask everyone to bring a stone that I can hold. Then Genny brings wine and seeds. We offer the wine to any guardian angels out there, then we breathe our intentions into the seeds and plant them in the ground. At one point, I lie down in the grass while my friends gather around me and put their hands gently on my shoulders, head, arms, and legs. They say beautiful, loving things about me. I am just supposed to lie there and receive, without saying anything.

It is uncomfortable and awkward and I keep wanting to get up and check to see if everyone is doing ok, if they need water or snacks or sunscreen, but I lie there obediently. I feel intuitively, irrationally, that learning to receive others' love and support is the same practice as learning to receive that I have a tumor. The alternative is to resist both. But resistance takes a lot of energy and I'd rather spend that energy on getting well. Acceptance is crucial to healing.

Eventually, I relax into their hands and the earth. I can smell the grass and feel the sun on my face. I say to myself, *I receive sunlight, I receive bird song, I receive the sound of dragonfly wings whirring overhead, and I receive my friends' gaze.* I don't try to say anything or guess what is going to happen next. I accept my life. I lie there and receive love.

13

Two nights later, we are walking around Boston with our parents and siblings. It feels like our wedding again. Our families have traveled all this way to support us. I feel like a bride, complete with the highs of being surrounded by love, and the lows of wanting everything to work out perfectly. Luckily, Aidan and Celia, my nephew and niece, put me at ease and make me laugh. Then my brothers take some of the pressure off by pouring affection on our kids. They arrange a great birthday party for Cole. They teach him to sail in Boston Harbor, buy him a skateboard, find cool places to try it, and let Hazel pick out the chocolate ice cream cake that we all share at dinner. While our families eat, Kurt and I go to meet with my doctor. The surgeries begin tomorrow.

We take a taxi to the hospital. The minute we step into the car and away from the laughter of my family, my mood changes. I stare out the window. I expect to see the world at a standstill. Instead, I see a woman buying flowers from an older man, a construction worker taking down a road sign, a child bouncing a soccer ball on his knee. Nothing has changed. But everything has changed for me. It surprises me that people can just go on with their lives when mine is going to end tomorrow.

"Am I the only one facing reality?" I ask Kurt. "Everyone says to me, "You've got this. But I don't feel like I have anything."

"No one knows how this is going to turn out. Not Dr. Al-Mefty. Not you."

"But what does it mean that I feel like I'm going to die?"

"Maybe that's just your mind responding to fear. It's not a *prediction* of what will happen," Kurt says firmly.

I try to process what Kurt has just said. My certainty that I'm going to die is a response, not a prediction. It feels like I know something others don't, but maybe it's just my mind trying to prepare for a complete unknown. I remind myself that there are plenty of people who have survived something like this and lived a long, long time after. There is no reason why I can't be one of them. "But, still," Fear reminds me, "The odds are not good."

"It is my job to tell you again about the risks," says Dr. Al-Mefty in a tiny examining room at the hospital. "This rare tumor cannot be cured. It can only be controlled. The more we remove, the better your chances are that it doesn't grow back bigger. But there are risks. It is wrapped around your brainstem and your throat. You may die. You may lose your voice, your ability to eat, and your ability to breathe, swallow, and speak on your own. There could be feeding tubes, a tracheotomy, and a mechanical voice box. Your tongue might not work again. Do you understand?"

"I understand," I say.

"You have a choice. I can go in and remove the tumor, as much as is safely possible. Or I can go in and remove the tumor, period. What do you choose?" Dr. Al-Mefty looks me right in the eyes when he asks this.

Sometimes, navigating this experience of having a brainstem tumor feels like there is no ground beneath my feet and the magnetic poles have shifted. I am paddling as hard as I can in a wide ocean, but the waves keep crashing hard on my head.

Other times, like now, it feels like I have immeasurable strength inside. I can't see it, but I can feel it: a deep, internal compass that I can rely on. It tells me what to do. It says again, *I choose brave over perfect.*

"Remove the tumor. All of it," I say.

Dr. Al-Mefty turns to look at Kurt. Kurt nods his approval.

"You deserve the best chance," Dr. Al-Mefty says, smiling.

I hold Kurt's hand. It feels steady and warm.

Back at the hotel, we tuck the kids into bed. I feel my heart break a little as I say goodnight. Then I dig through my suitcase to find the letter I wrote to Hazel. I've already given Kurt and Cole their letters to read when they are ready.

"You know that it's always been easier for me to say how I feel in writing," I say when I give Hazel's letter to Kurt.

"Is it for her now, or later, when she's a little older?" He asks.

"For later. I wrote it thinking, What do I wish I had known as a young woman? But it was tough to write. I kept wondering, What do I tell her and what do I let her figure out on her own?"

"Don't you think she needs to figure out *everything* on her own?" Kurt asks, teasing me a little.

"Maybe, but I'm way too controlling for that," I say.

"Don't worry. I won't need to give her the letter. You'll be around to give it to her yourself," he says with such confidence that, for a second, I dare to believe him.

My mind travels to the Pacific Ocean, twenty years earlier.

"Remember when we met, and I asked you about the magnetic poles switching?" I ask.

"I remember," Kurt says.

"I was really scared about losing north."

"How do you feel now?" he asks.

"Like you said, we need to get lost to change the way we look at things. I think I am going to be alright through these surgeries. We are all going to be okay. Maybe we have to look south to find north," I say, before drifting off to sleep.

⟶⟵

Dear Hazel,

You are ten years old as I write this letter, which is meant for you to read as a young woman. This is your map to self. This is your map to safety. At ten, you talk to flowers, pose questions to the moon, go on brave adventures, and make up songs. The other night you sang a song you wrote, "I know that everyone has a star, but I don't know which is mine." Your lyrics are often about finding your way. When you are lost, unfold this letter and find yourself. Find me, too, holding your hand and your heart.

One morning in June, you curled next to me, lifted my arm over your tiny shoulders, and we snuggled deep into our gray couch. It's then that we talked about the tumor.

"Do you understand that I may not have much time in this life?" I asked.

"Yes, but it doesn't matter," you said.

"Why?"

"Because I can't tell time!" you said with a straight face.

Then I laughed.

"Why are you laughing?" you asked.

"Because I love you," I said.

When you were born, you were bald and pink and curled up like a smooth-skinned armadillo. Yet I thought you were absolutely beautiful. I spent hours watching your lips, stroking your fingers, counting your toes. It was as if I could see and touch my own heart outside of my body; it was as if I could see and touch joy itself when holding you. And yet I was quickly filled with the fear that something might happen to you. I would wake up with horrible thoughts and feelings of grief even though nothing had happened.

When you began to sleep in your own room, I needed to know if you were breathing, but I didn't want to wake you by opening the old, creaky door to your bedroom. In the middle of the night, I would walk outside the house in my nightgown and take steps through the snow to get to your window, just to watch your chest rise and fall through the glass. Then back through the snow and into the house, only to repeat the vigil in the snow two hours later. My love for you has always been like a long exhale of joy, interrupted by short, sharp inhales of fear.

Mostly, I feared that I was not good enough. You may feel that way sometimes, like you are not good enough. Just ask women of all ages for their stories. You will hear the constellations of suffering and beauty that make up who we are.

You may also feel as though there is something wrong with you, because you can't keep up with the world's expectations. There is nothing wrong with you. When you question your worth, remember: you were born worthy. It is not something you need to earn or prove. Your value is like my love for you; it is in flash-flood mode all the time, with no banks or limits.

I want to rebel against the idea that our bodies are not already perfect, as they are. What if we praised our eyes, lips, fingers and toes, bones, shoulders, and muscles for all of their genius? What if we admired them the way we admire other natural bodies like the sun, moon, and stars?

At ten, you are in love with your body: the strength and speed of your legs, the joys of your flexibility, the power and grace of your muscles. Soon, you may think your body is something to hide and to hate. Listen. Your body is perfect as it is. You have your Nana's angular legs and arms, your Grandma's nose and wavy hair, my deep-set eyes and fair skin, and your own full lips and mouth. Your body is your connection to me, to your grandmothers, and to women around the world. It is the home of the umbilical cord and the womb.

When I was a little older than you, I was embarrassed that I didn't yet have my period. Then, when I finally got it, I was ashamed of my body. I wore baggy clothes to hide my shape, and I spat at my reflection in the mirror in disgust. When you get your period, celebrate. I'm serious. Your period may be annoying, but it is not shameful. By shedding the lining of your uterus once a month and building a fresh one, your body is teaching you to let go of what does not serve you. Your body is powerful and magnificent.

Becoming a woman is not just about your body changing; it is the process of discovering who you are by listening to your inner voice. Becoming a woman is growing brave enough to express yourself, even when you are afraid.

I believe it begins by trusting that your contribution, no matter how small, matters.

Sometimes being brave means to be bold, but sometimes it means to be vulnerable. Sometimes it means to forge ahead, other times it means to be still. Sometimes it means to fight, other times, being brave means to let go. What it means to be brave will change as you change.

"Mama, will my voice change when I grow up?" You asked me the other day. I guess you had heard that your brother's voice will soon crack and deepen.

"No, no. Your voice will always stay the same," I said dismissively.

But that's not true. If you think about your voice as the instrument with which you author your life, and not just the physical sounds that come out of your throat, then it will definitely change, and it will get lost, and you will find it again. You will lose it when you try to please everyone. To find your voice again, remember what you loved to do when you were nine or ten years old, before others' voices mattered more to you than your own.

In case you've forgotten, you spent whole afternoons climbing trees, singing songs you created, and inventing elaborate treasure hunts. What if you devoted a day to no one but yourself and nature? And instead of trying to reach a summit, you explored around you, with bravery, curiosity, and imagination? Do what feels good, despite your fear saying, *You will disappoint everyone and go broke*. Slowly, through a daily practice of being brave, your fear will get bored and shut up, while your unique voice gets louder and clearer.

I can't help but make a connection between our mutual love of treasure hunts and this crazy experience called life. How can it be that we can love these hunts so much, but be uncomfortable facing big uncertainties in life such as *Will I find love? My purpose? A way to save the world?* It's easy to get scared into thinking there isn't a next clue. But I'm here to tell you that there will always be a next clue and you will always find it.

If you live like that, with bravery and trust, then life becomes one big treasure hunt, an adventurous game that is our privilege to play.

I have no solid footing to tell you that you will never be left alone, or that your worth will always be recognized by others. To the little girl inside me, nothing is more murky than my value. Yet nothing is more clear to me than your value. You are powerful and you belong here.

When you feel like a dancer without a floor, or a tree without roots, know that I am with you. I am as much a part of you as your fingers, your toes, your beating heart, your wild instincts, your breath. Feel me listening to you, holding you, and giving you a loud, standing ovation.

Love,
Mama

Facing the Storm

When a huge storm of change and uncertainty approaches, it's almost impossible to know how to respond. If we are still standing, call it a success. But then what? We can resist the challenge before us or we can accept it and change the only thing in our control: our response. Once we see the problem before us as necessary, uncomfortable, but also potentially transformative, the way forward becomes clear. We don't have to know what to do before we begin. We only have to be open and curious.

Consider the ways that helped me to put one foot in front of the other:

- *Get quiet and be alone.* Find a safe space to listen to your fears and your inner strength.

- *Feel all of your feelings.* Name them (truck on my chest, pit in my belly, rock on my shoulders). My favorite is "red-hot rage in my throat." I kick trash cans and slam doors; the more you give yourself permission to feel *all* emotions, the more capacity you'll have to feel joy.

- *Separate pain from suffering.* Pain is real. It is loss, sickness, injury, and heartbreak. Suffering is what we do to ourselves with our habit of worrying and imagining worst-case scenarios. Don't add suffering to pain. There is already too much suffering in the world as it is. Decide to choose joy over fear.

- *Trust.* Remember times when things worked out, despite the odds. Your wallet was returned to you. The car didn't run out of gas. You found somewhere else to live. The dog came home. The more you accept that the universe has your back, and that you are not in control, the easier a challenge becomes. You still work hard, get help from others, and learn from mistakes, but then lie back and float. The water will hold you.

- *Come up with a mantra.* Repeat it to yourself (all will be well, brave over perfect, temporary pain, long-term gain, the best is yet to come). Say it often, especially before each step forward, the same way you pause to make a wish before blowing out birthday candles.

- *Tell your community.* You can tell one trusted person at a time, or all at once. You never know who can help. I believe this is why we're here: to walk through hard times together.

- *Create a list of things that make you feel light, supported, and strong.* Don't keep the list in a drawer. Pick the first thing on the list and ask someone for help with it. Or, give the list to a trusted friend and have that person do the asking until you're ready to do it yourself. (On my list, I included things that didn't help such as, "Don't ask me questions." You could add, "Don't give me advice," or "Please only visit if you fold laundry.")

- *Gratitude is the guardian of happiness.* Each day, name one thing that makes you feel grateful. Avoid general ones, like "my life." Use your five senses and get specific. "I'm grateful for the sound of rain on the roof." Do this to develop a lens of positivity and you'll notice more things to be thankful for each day.

- *Surround yourself with beauty and laughter.* For me, that means flowers and little kids. Whatever it is for you, make it a priority.

PART III

THE FASTEST WAY TO A STRONG VOICE

14

Moments before surgery, my body feels like it is ringing inside the bells at Notre-Dame Cathedral in Paris. But it is just the metal coils in the MRI vibrating loudly during pre-operative tests. I let the sound ring this question out of me:

If you come out of these surgeries unharmed, with a full life ahead of you, how are you going to live? Will you do anything differently?

Everyone has their way of trying to answer the big questions in their lives. Talking to friends and mentors is one way. My way is to write. I write to know what I am thinking. I write to understand what I am feeling. I write to remember and to re-member, to put myself back together one piece at a time.

What follows are excerpts from my journal. SV = Small Victory. I recorded one each day.

8.1.16 *SV: I don't back out of the operations*

Surgery day. We wake up at 3:30 a.m. to walk to the hospital. The kids are still sleeping. I kiss them on their foreheads goodbye. My parents and brothers are in the lobby of the hotel, awake to see us off. A few hugs and it's time to go. "You're as strong as a streetcar," my dad calls to me as I walk down the dark sidewalk. I raise my fist in the air, letting him know I hear him.

It's still dark outside, but warm enough that I am in a t-shirt and shorts. I feel like I am about to begin a big running race. I am up early, walking to the start. Everything I need is in this little plastic bag that I carry: a change of clothes; the book of letters from my students;

photographs of my parents, my brothers, and Kurt with the kids; plus my journal.

On the way to the hospital, I bang on the locked doors of a church, then try to pry them open. I want to go in and light a candle. Kurt points out that it's not a church, but an apartment building that used to be a church. We run to hide in the bushes in case we've woken someone up. We buckle over, laughing.

Luckily, there is a small chapel in the hospital. While Kurt waits for them to call my name in the pre-operative area, I find the small, carpeted sanctuary. There is not much there: a few chairs, a makeshift altar with three battery-powered candles, a bulletin board covered in requests for help. "Please bring Mommy home today," says one. This reminds me that I have a prayer I want to say. I found it one day after yoga class when my teacher said to me out of the blue, "Let me hear your prayer."

"My what?"

"Everybody prays when they are in trouble," she smiles, knowingly.

"Please let me live. Please let me be here to help my children grow," I say, slightly embarrassed.

"Sounds like begging to me. There is nothing more powerful than a woman, especially a mother, who is in need. Try again. Claim the power you have."

I take a deep breath and try again, "I accept this challenge. But now I need you in my corner. I will survive and be with my children. I will grow old with my husband. I will live and give back to the world. Be with me."

"That's more like it!" she laughs.

Now in the hospital chapel, I kneel down and close my eyes. I begin, "I accept this challenge…"

Kurt walks in just as I am finishing my prayer, "Ready?" he asks.

"Ready," I say, but my voice shakes.

8.2.16 Cole's Birthday. He is thirteen today. *SV: survive thirty-six hours of surgery*

I wake up in the Intensive Care Unit. I can't talk—my throat feels like I have swallowed a truck. I can't swallow. Is this normal?

Dr. Al-Mefty comes in and tells me Kurt has been sitting in the waiting room for thirty-six hours. The kids are with their grandparents. I want to ask if it's over.

"It's done," says my doctor, reading my mind.

"Rest now."

I wake up again because my hip hurts. I point to it and play charades with one of my surgeons, Dr. Omar Arnaout, to ask why.

"Sorry," says Dr. Arnaout. "We had to take part of your hip to put in your neck. The tumor had eroded a lot of bone on your cervical spine."

My back hurts.

"Sorry," says Dr. Arnaout. "We had to take a rib, too."

My stomach hurts.

"Oh yeah," says my doctor. "We needed some fat to stick the bones together and rebuild your spine. Your mother offered to donate some fat. But we went with yours instead."

I want to ask, "Will I speak again?" but no sound comes out of my throat. Dr. Arnaout doesn't understand.

"Rest," he says.

8.3.16 *SV: breathing on my own*

Today, some of the finest neurosurgeons at Harvard, Mass General, Brigham Women's Hospital, and Dana Farber Cancer Center gathered together to review my case.

Can the patient breathe on her own?	Yes.
Can she see? Hear? Taste?	Yes. Yes. Yes.
Can she think clearly on her own?	Yes.
Can she move her arms and legs?	Yes.
Can she talk?	We don't know yet.

8.4.16 *SV: first time standing up*

I notice faces of everyone I have ever known appearing and disappearing before my eyes. I see my mother's face in the stream of light coming through the door, my father's face on the TV monitor, the smile of a former student in the white sheet tucked over my arms, the flowing hair of a friend in the curtains, kisses blown to me from my nieces and nephews from the ceiling tiles.

Some say your life flashes before your eyes at the end, but this is not what I imagined. The faces are like floating candles on a raft, carrying me safely to shore over a deep lake. And of course, there is the explanation that I am heavily medicated; I can label these images hallucinations and call it a day. But these faces are so clear and so specific, I can't dismiss them so easily.

When the music of my inhales and exhales threatened to fade away to nothing and I felt the last page of the book of my life between my thumb and forefinger, I saw the faces of family and friends. I saw everyone who carried me toward safety with positive thoughts and prayers, lit candles, and ceremonies. I believe they had a hand in this great outcome.

8.5.16 *SV: moved out of the ICU*

The nurses in the ICU call me the "Thumbs-Up Girl." I can't speak, so I use my hands to talk.

"You ok?" I give them the thumbs up.

"How are the pain meds?" Thumbs up.

"So they're good then?"

I shake my head no. I give the thumbs up and then push it up into the air. And up. And up. "More meds!" I am trying to say.

8.6.16 *SV: first solid food: two bites of jello*

The kids are here. Our friends Faith and John bring them to the hospital. This is the first time that they'll see me since the surgeries. *Will they love me like this?* Cole walks in the room first. He looks taller, more grown-up. He comes right up to me and holds my hand. Hazel pauses before coming all the way into the room. She stands at the foot of the hospital bed and says sadly, "You don't look like my Mama."

My heart breaks a little.

8.7.16 *SV: brushed my teeth*

I'm frustrated and sad. My head is wrapped in a tight bandage to prevent spinal fluid from leaking out. My neck is locked in a collar to protect the fusion. I can't speak. I go to write and my right arm throbs with nerve pain. It feels like I have an electric eel surging through me. I try to go on Facebook and yet all I see are people having summertime fun while I lie here. My brother and friends are dancing at a rock concert and I can't even stand up on my own. Read? Can't concentrate. Walk? Too unsteady. Watch TV? Hurts my head. The room I'm in smells like urine and jello. The machines I'm attached to beep constantly. If I move too far away from them, a screeching alarm sounds. I'm just trying to get closer to the window. I want to see a tree. Just one tree. Something green. It's almost night again. I hate nighttime. While others sleep, I sit up in pain. When I lie down, I stop breathing. *Is this my life?*

8.8.16 Kurt's Birthday. *SV: picked up a pen and wrote*

I am discharged from the hospital. It's scary to be away from nurses and immediate care, but it is deliciously quiet. We are renting a home from a friend of a friend in a quiet suburb of Boston. There are trees swaying outside my open window. The air smells like fresh-cut grass. My blood pressure dropped fifty millimeters within hours of leaving the hospital. Now I'm watching Kurt sleep. He is lying on top of the covers, ready to wake up and help me at any moment. I smile at the way he always hooks his thumbs into the top of his boxers. Today is his birthday. I find a pen.

For Kurt on his birthday, a poem:

> At midnight, my husband is awake,
>   his hands moving gently,
>   measuring out my medications.
> At 2 a.m., he makes three trips up the stairs
> to hand me water, then a straw that bends,
>   then potatoes and chicken, mashed
>   into Skittle-sized pieces with a spoon.
>   Now it's 4 a.m. and he is awake again,

holds my hand as we walk in the dark
because I can't sleep.
We step under a giant cottonwood tree
and touch its braided bark.
I have been restless my whole life,
running up summits to see
what shiny beauty is on the other side,
but the beauty I see now is everywhere,
especially in the simple hand gestures of this man.
He finds a loose strand of my hair
tucks it neatly behind my head bandage,
holds my head in his hands,
and kisses me.

8.9.16 *SV: had stitches removed*

A summer storm. I am up at 2:30 a.m., watching the lightning illuminate the room in bright bursts, and listening to the thunder explode while the rain streams in through the open windows. I can't sleep. They say anger is the second stage of grief. So far, I have been thinking, *anger is not my issue.* Until tonight. Tonight, I start to cry. I feel so angry that I don't have a voice. I feel so angry that there are women around the world who never have a voice. I feel angry that my family has to help me put on my socks and feed me. Then I groan and grit my teeth and growl out all my anger and frustration and sadness. I think of Hazel and how she didn't want to come near me. I hear her words echoing in my heart, "You don't look like my Mama." I feel anger that she is repulsed by me and anger that I can't hold her tight without it hurting my neck. It's all coming out now. I sit and cry and growl.

8.10.16 *SV: first bath*

Not having a voice is lonely. In front of the bathroom mirror, I open my mouth, stick out my tongue. The left side of it is numb and wavy, like ribbon candy. The doctors say the nerves will come back eventually. For now, I can't move the right side of my tongue or feel it. There is also some damage to my vocal cords. I say to the mirror, as loud as I can, "Good morning!" What comes out is nothing more than a squeaky whisper. In the doorway, I shout Kurt's name. He is on the other side of the bed, no more than ten feet away from me. He keeps folding the laundry. He cannot hear me. *So this is the taste of voicelessness: bitter isolation, acidic futility, burning determination.* I took my voice for granted. Never again.

8.11.16 *SV: slept for three hours in a row!*

What's toughest for me is trying to figure out how to be me, only different. I hear Cole playing basketball outside alone and I can't join him. I can't even walk on my own. *How do I play with our children when they want to play ball and do things that I can't do?*

8.12.16 *SV: first time wearing clothes*

My childhood friends travel hundreds, even thousands, of miles to come see me. Natasha is here visiting now. Teza was here last week. Alli is coming soon. Three reasons to be grateful.

8.13.16 *SV: first time walking without holding someone's hand*

Kurt and I have a fight. The car we are borrowing breaks down on the way to the hospital. "Should we roll it and jump start it? Should we call a tow truck?" I ask in breathy, stuttered bursts. Kurt says, "Every time you ask a question, you hand over responsibility to me. And it feels like you don't have confidence in me." It's a communication problem; I ask questions to feel like I am brainstorming in the moment and we are working together.

He says, "Can't you just say, 'You've got this. I know you've dealt with cars before; you'll figure this out?'" What he needs is to feel like I know him. He doesn't need brainstorming.

So I cry and pull away from him. I think, *How can you scold me right now for something I did in a stressful moment on the way to the hospital? How can you tell me to just keep saying, "I know you've got this," when that means handing over one more aspect of a life that I have less and less control of every day?*

I say, "I need to feel empowered instead of powerless and disengaged. I engage by asking questions."

"I know. It's just that I need to feel like you have confidence in me."

What I want to hear now is "All will be well." And then I realize that's exactly what Kurt needs too. He needs someone to tell him "All will be well" instead of all of us leaning on him to fix all that feels broken.

8.14.16 *SV: gave myself shots for thinning blood clots in my legs from surgery*

We finally find out the diagnosis of the tumor. It is a rare form of cancer that cannot be cured, but it can be controlled. Nothing has changed. We still don't want to talk with others about the kind of tumor it is. And we refuse to attach ourselves to a prognosis based on averages. We want to focus on my particular experience. Another way to use my voice is to find a grounded stillness in what I think is true, which is that I will recover fully. I prefer to stay quiet than to drown my friends in information about the tumor.

Others use the language of "fighting" and "beating" a disease. *I am a fighter. I will win this war.* But it's not working for me. It makes me anxious. *I should do more to beat this thing. I am not tough enough because the disease is still there. I must be weak.* So, I am trying a different angle.

Instead of fighting, I'm practicing the uncomfortable art of embracing my condition. *Can I accept the tumor and see it as a catalyst for change in my life? Can I believe that the best is yet to come?* I want to accept my reality at the same time that I believe that it's not my time to leave the planet. I have a lot to give.

8.15.16 *SV: off all pain medication*

Our first family outing to a nearby park. In the car on the way there, Hazel is sitting behind me. She has a perfect view of the scars on my neck and skull. She sings loudly,

> "Mama's scars are gro-o-o-o-dy,
> But I don't want to say anything mean,
> So I'll just turn my head,
> Close my eyes, and
> Hope I don't see them!"

Her song is honest, and it helps break the tension. We all burst into laughter.

8.16.16 *SV: took off neck brace for one hour*

Dr. Chi, the surgeon who rebuilt my spine, is staring at an X-ray of my neck and skull.

"Everything looks good. Just don't run."

"What do you mean? No running for how long? A month?" I ask. I feel taken aback, and then embarrassed, as if I sound ungrateful.

"Maybe never. The impact of running is not good for you."

"What's the danger?" I assume he's exaggerating. I'm asking for details so I can find a way out of this death sentence for my life as a runner.

"Your head is held on with metal rods and screws. You risk loosening or breaking the hardware. One danger is that you become paralyzed."

"Oh," I say. But what I feel is, *There is no way out.*

That night, we take the kids to see the Disney movie, *Pete's Dragon.* The movie isn't great, but it isn't terrible either. For two hours, I allow myself to feel like I am running through the woods like the hero of the movie. When the lights come up and I realize that I can't run, that I can barely walk, I crumble in tears. It isn't a dream, I really am "compromised" and am going to be limited for a long, long time. Kurt sees me crying and he understands; he starts to cry too. When a couple walks by and gives us a look of concern, I hear Kurt say, "Emotional movie, wasn't it?"

8.17.16 *SV: went down and up the stairs alone*

The doctors are talking about inserting a gastric feeding tube directly into my stomach. There is concern about my difficulty swallowing. I am not gaining weight. Now, at one hundred pounds, I don't have much energy. My throat is damaged. And I still don't have a voice. When I hear the words "feeding tube," I immediately start planning for the Olympics of swallowing. I will smash the world record for excellent barium swallow test results and they will never talk to me again about feeding tubes.

I meet a speech therapist in her tiny, cramped office, which was decorated in joyful artwork with a colorful quilt on the wall, made by some of her patients. She is energetic, and a little too supportive for my taste. She asks me to swallow water. I take a sip. She claps her hands together, and exclaims, "Good job!" It's nice, but it feels undeserved. "You're ready for applesauce," she says with an encouraging smile.

"Oh boy," I say. I think, *At this rate, I'm doomed. They may as well order the feeding tube now.*

"What can I do to train my throat to swallow better?"

"It's not your throat, really. The right side of your tongue is paralyzed. That side can't help usher food down. You just need to slow way down."

"What about my voice? What's wrong with it?" I ask.

"You have lost some strength and balance. Working optimally, vocal cords vibrate fast. For women, they open and close at a rate of 180 to 220 cycles per second. Yours are slower. That's why it sounds like you are whispering. Air is passing over the cords, but they are not vibrating fast enough to make strong sounds. But that's all. I don't see permanent damage."

"Can I do anything to bring my voice back faster?"

"Your full-time job now is recovering. Rest. Be patient."

"Is it psychological?" I ask, nervously.

"No. Vocal cords are not like guitar strings. They are sensitive to tension. In this case, working harder will make them worse. The fastest way to a strong voice is to relax," she says firmly. Then she smiles, touches my shoulder with her hand, and sends me on my way.

I absorb the lesson: the way to a clear, powerful voice is to do less. Try "easy" instead of try hard. *Can I really get stronger by being me, by doing nothing?*

15

August 18, 2016

I'm back in that moment in bed, wondering, *Who am I?* I am not a wife, not a mother, not a leader, not an athlete. I am a lump in a bed. I can't even help my daughter make breakfast. The old way of constantly doing and moving isn't available. I can't just get up and make myself busy. *Plus, didn't the old way put me in this bed?* The late-morning sun feels hotter than usual. I feel pinned to the sheets. I can't reach the window blind to pull it down, to make the pain stop.

I should feel grateful. I am alive. I am out of the hospital. But it feels forced. I sit in bed, propped up by a dozen pillows, barely able to move. I still can't speak above a whisper. Fear says, "You're not getting better fast enough." I constantly think I feel wet spinal fluid dripping down my neck. I can't sleep. I can't lie down without my neck brace blocking my airway. I can't swallow anything larger than a pea. I can't walk on my own. I can't run now, or ever again.

I have always identified with the hero role. I am out there, in the adventure, making things happen. I can push through anything. But there are consequences to pushing, striving, fixing, saving everything and everyone. I put so much pressure on myself that I get sick. This time, my health isn't just telling me to slow down. It's telling me to transform completely. *How many times do I have to learn this lesson?*

Kurt comes to check on me. He gives me my medications and examines the back of my head bandage.

"I feel like a loser lying here, doing nothing," I whisper.

"You are doing something; you're healing," Kurt says. I am not convinced.

"Give me a mountain to climb, a raging river to cross, monsters with knives to fight. Please just don't make me lie still," I beg him. Kurt ignores me. He opens the window to let in some fresh air, pulls the blind down, gives me a kiss, and heads back downstairs to take care of our kids. As soon as he opens the window, a dragonfly soars into the room. It patrols the perimeter of my bed. I can hear the tiny whirr of its wings.

One summer in my twenties, I became fascinated by metamorphosis. I was in graduate school and a little lost; I felt like a messed-up kid in an adult world. I wanted to know what I needed to do to become a "real" grown-up. I studied the life cycles of insects obsessively, spending long days at the pond near where I was living. Before, I thought that a caterpillar went into a cocoon and came out with wings as a butterfly. I didn't know that a caterpillar dissolves completely inside that chrysalis until it is nothing but green liquid. This comforts me to remember. *No wonder transformation is uncomfortable.* In the process of becoming someone new, I have to dissolve first.

One day that summer, I found a large dragonfly nymph in the pond and brought it home with me. Dragonflies have a different transformation process than butterflies; they begin as ugly-looking insects under water before hatching into flying jewels. I wanted to catch it in the act of changing, so I put my nymph in a glass cookie jar full of pond water. I thought for sure it would morph momentarily, based on its size. I ended up feeding it tadpoles *for weeks* while it stared at me from its cookie jar on the kitchen table. I kept looking for signs that the dragonfly was ready to bust out of its old self to become new. But the nymph didn't do anything. *How did it learn to fly?*

Then one morning, it crawled out of the water to breathe air for the first time. It looked like it was in pain. It was limp, wet, and clutching the top of the jar. Then it slowly gained color and strength. I opened the front door, and it flew away on its own. Its brand-new wings looked like tiny stained glass windows. I was amazed; a water creature that eats tadpoles can now fly over thirty miles an hour! I couldn't believe that it didn't do anything to cause its transformation. It just happened one day. Apparently, a wingless, watery dragonfly already contains everything it needs to fly when it's born.

What is inside me? I don't know. I feel as though I lost the map to myself one piece at a time, as I let others' voices tell me who I was. And, I never stopped moving long enough to listen to my own inner voice. I was so busy looking outside, racking up achievements, that I never looked inside. The dragonfly that flew in this window reminds me that transformation is not something I have to make happen. It's something I *allow* to happen.

How would I act if I believed that everything I need is with me right now? Would I lie still and just be, if I knew that I was already perfect?

16

When Mom arrives in Boston to help me recover, she sets down her hot pink bag in my room and declares, "I don't cook. I don't do dishes. Never have. Never will." I sigh, remembering that caregiving is not my mother's strongest skill. At seventy-five years old, she is unconventional and adventurous. I appreciate her and love her deeply, but that's never stopped me from wanting Mom to be different.

When I was young, I wanted a mother who was sweet and nurturing, who baked cookies, who drove me places, and who welcomed my friends with cheerful holiday decorations. What I got was a mother who raised us well, but without coddling, and who cooked so rarely that she kept a heavy chair in front of our oven door. On Halloween, she turned off the lights and left a bowl of toothbrushes on the front step. At Christmas, she hung a tangled strand of lights on a house plant and called it a day. When I got my driver's license, she traded our car for a painting.

As a child, I yelled, "Why can't you be more like other moms? A mom who makes dinner, vacuums, and who doesn't forget to pick her kids up from summer camp!"

"We care about different things, that's all," she'd respond. "I'd rather be out there, in the world, than cooking or cleaning up your messes. And I didn't forget you, I just got the day wrong on my calendar."

"*Twice*," I point out.

At night, I prayed for a different mother. I thought mine was doing it wrong. I didn't see that she was modeling authenticity for me. Her inner voice has always been clear and strong. *Be yourself!* Her actions screamed. I just kept missing the memo. *Can I learn the message now?*

My favorite picture book as a child was *Are You My Mother?*, a book about a bird who falls out of its nest and goes looking for its mother, asking the cow, the hen, even a bulldozer, "Are you my mother?" The book is an inside joke between Mom and me, because I always felt so different from her. As a teenager, I was a hippie girl and she was more of a Spice Girl. I lay on the floor and listened to Bob Dylan while she moonwalked to Michael Jackson. She was messy and I organized everything. I wanted to fit in; she wanted to stand out. She seemed to be carefree. I worried constantly about the state of the world. She held firm, clear boundaries; I ran ragged trying to keep everyone happy.

When I read that the legendary folk singer, Joni Mitchell, gave up a daughter about my age for adoption, I fantasized that Joni was my real mother. I imagined the warm embrace when we would finally meet, and the cover story that would run in the newspaper with the headline, "Mother and Child Reunion."

Now that I am a mother, I am sure my children want me to be different, too. It comes with the territory. I can't cook. I write stories, often about them. And when they have a project due in school, it becomes the target of my anxious perfectionism. They have legitimate complaints. Still, I believe that the mother we get and the mother we want is the original line between fact and fiction, reality and fantasy.

In Boston, Mom is sure that the best way for me to heal is to watch the Olympic tennis matches on TV. Mom is fanatical about tennis. She yells at the screen, jumps out of her seat during a great rally, and spills popcorn all over me when a player makes an unlikely return shot. These moments remind me of my childhood.

For my sixteenth birthday, Mom took me to see the tennis greats Steffi Graf and Martina Navratilova. When Steffi won, I assumed it was time to go home. Mom had a different idea.

"Quick!" she said. "Steffi's signing autographs!" At courtside, Mom pushed me through a crowd of wild and enthusiastic tennis fans.

"It's her birthday. Let her through." Mom pushed harder, smiling brightly at her fellow fans.

"What's your name?" Steffi Graf asked me as she signed my poster.

"Marilyn! Her name is Marilyn!" Mom shouted from the back of the crowd. When we finally left with *her* signed poster, Mom laughed. This is the thing about my mother: she can laugh at herself easily, joyfully.

When I became a wife and a mother, I thought that if I acted a little less myself and more polished and perfect like I imagined other women to be, my husband would stay and my kids would be happy. I traded my uniqueness for convention. I thought, *I should read less and cook more. I should yell less and smile more. I should make less mess and clean more.* I lost track of who I was and what my voice sounded like free of "shoulds."

I worked to maintain my status as the good daughter, the good wife, the good worker, the good mother. I managed others' needs and feelings to the detriment of my own to the point where, when Kurt asked me one day, "What do you need?" I had nothing to say. I had no idea.

Now, with Mom here to "take care of me," I am learning that there is a connection between not accepting Mom and not accepting myself for who we are. Instead of wishing Mom were different, I am trying to appreciate my mother for who she is. I am also trying to appreciate myself for who I am. We are more similar than I think. And she knows me so well.

Here in Boston, when I am tired, she knows to take my phone away and guard my door for privacy. Before I can even tell her that I am hungry, she makes me instant oatmeal and only partially destroys the stovetop. When I am restless and cranky, she straps on her squeaky tennis shoes and leads me out the door. She is protective as we walk slowly along the bike path. She doesn't want me to turn too quickly and hurt my neck.

"A bunny!" she shouts. "But don't look!"

Best of all, she plays with the kids while I sleep. Our kids love their Nana, even if she does always send them back to the start when they play "Sorry!" because she is one-hundred-percent herself. Mom being here is teaching me that being unapologetically myself, complete with scars and a stiff neck, is the greatest gift I can give my children.

17

Dr. Al-Mefty gives me some unexpected news during a routine follow-up appointment. There are two other surgeons in the examining room with us at the neurological center of Brigham and Women's hospital. The surgeons touch my head, my neck, and my arms. They unwrap and rewrap my head bandage. Then they talk among themselves while I sit in a hospital gown, on a cold table, and Kurt sits in a chair near the door. Suddenly, all three stop talking and look at me. Dr. Al-Mefty speaks first.

"What I am needing to tell you is this; there is a piece of tumor on your spine. It is sitting on C5. It's ok, small. I'll take it out, you will be fine."

"You missed a piece and now I need more surgery? Is that what you are saying?" I don't intend to be rude; I am genuinely trying to understand.

Dr. Chi weighs in, looking at Dr. Al-Mefty, not at me. "We better go in now, before the neck fusion sets too much. As is, we'll have to take apart the hardware in there and rebuild."

"But we don't know. It is small. Radiation may take care of it," responds Dr. Al-Mefty.

"The standard treatment is surgery, then radiation. Remember, the future is a question of control not cure. A controlled tumor is one that is quiet and dormant, not gone," offers Dr. Arnaout.

"How much radiation?" I ask.

"I don't know. Two, three months? As soon as possible," says Dr. Al-Mefty.

"Think of surgery and radiation like weed control. First you pull out the weeds you can see, which we did. But if you stop there, you leave a bit of root or a long-dormant seed buried in the soil and a new weed can sprout. Radiation zaps the roots of the tumor and the bone from where it originated," Dr. Arnaout explains. We listen. Kurt nods.

"What can I do?" I ask, fighting back tears.

"Nothing. Rest. We'll talk to the radiation oncologist and let you know in a few days if you need surgery and just how much radiation to expect."

I feel like I'm falling down a dark, deep hole. There are no sounds except someone shouting from above, *More tumor! More surgery! Radiation immediately!* I knew I needed radiation, but I didn't know I needed to start now. And I never expected to need more surgery. I thought I could go home soon. Kurt drives us back to the rental house. I don't remember the drive, the August heat in the air, or the stop he made to get gas for the car. Fear is too busy shouting at me, "They should have done the full-spine scan earlier; they might have seen it. Why didn't you speak up then?" *I don't want to go back under the knife. I don't want there to be more tumor. I want to go home.*

There is nothing we can do but wait. In the house we are renting, I turn on the TV. The only thing on is news about the race for the presidency of the United States. I try not to watch, but I can't help it; I am drawn to the awful mess of it. I do not like the direction the country is going in. I want to grab the steering wheel and turn us in a more civil, generous, and inclusive direction. Instead, I sit here in bed and watch a man say racist, sexist things and gain momentum for the highest leadership position in the country, possibly the world. I am in disbelief. I definitely want things to turn out differently. How can a man who calls women "fat pigs," Mexicans "rapists," and Muslims "terrorists" become president? It makes me feel crazy and helpless. The guy who points his hand like a gun into the crowd and says, "I could shoot people and I wouldn't lose voters," is going to make decisions that affect our planet? The man who says that he wants to bring back "waterboarding and a hell of a lot worse than waterboarding" could be the next leader of the "free" world? I cannot let go. I need this election to turn out differently.

I try to read. Lately, I am reading books on how to face adversity without feeling anxious and panicky. Each author insists that I must surrender to what is and let go of control. Ajahn Chah, a Buddhist teacher says, "If you let go a little, you will have a little happiness. If you let go a lot, you will have a lot of happiness. If you let go completely, you will be completely happy."

He is not a mother, I remind myself. Letting go feels like giving up. The word surrender conjures up images of an exhausted, desperate soldier waving the white flag. That's not me. I don't give up. I can't even let go of my breath when I exhale, and I resist letting go of the words in any run-on sentence. I like being in control. I make things happen through will and perseverance.

I reach out to Michael, my therapist back in Colorado. He is a cancer survivor. I can't speak above a whisper, so I write a text message, "They say I need more surgery and a lot of radiation. I hope it's not true. I hope it's a mistake. Maybe we don't need to talk. Maybe just send me hope."

He texts me right back. It's a funny, modern kind of therapy. I imagine him taking his phone outside and sitting on the hillside above his office, one of my favorite spots in Boulder. I used to run there and see deer bedding down in the grass, foxes running ahead of me like red arrows, and a pair of Cooper's hawks nesting from the top of a ponderosa pine.

"Beware of hope," writes Michael. "You can't feel at peace if what you hope for is not happening. "I hope I don't need more surgery" quickly becomes "I'll only be happy if I don't need more surgery." Hope is clinging to a cure. That's a miserable way to live."

"K. What is the alternative?" I ask.

"Faith. Trust in life. Have faith that no matter what, you are safe, and your family is safe."

"But isn't that like saying, Ok, Universe, you're in charge, cut me up and kill me if you must?"

"No. You can still visualize that you are healthy and strong in the future. Positive visualization helps. But, you're not in charge. When you surrender to life and what is, you feel a lot more peace."

"I don't like the word surrender. It's too scary for me."

"Is there another word that works for you?" Michael asks.

"I don't know. But are you saying that if a doctor told you tomorrow that you were going to die in a few months, you would just accept that and trust that all will turn out well?"

"They did say that to me. Several doctors told me I only had weeks to live. I accepted their opinions as one piece, but not the whole story."

"But when I try that, I feel naïve, like I am not facing facts."

"What about the fact that countless people like you were told they only had days to live and then went on to have long, healthy lives?"

"I need to meet some of those people."

"You're texting one right now," Michael reminds me. "Can you remember a time that you wanted something, but it wasn't until you let it go, that you got it?"

"Sure. A high school crush. But by the time he liked me, I didn't care anymore."

"He was probably drawn to that less desperate energy! Ok. Now. Think of a time in your life when you surrendered to the unknown and there was a positive outcome. Do you have one?"

"I'm thinking…Got one. When I married Kurt. I can honestly say that life chose him for me."

"And life chose this tumor for you. But you can't say yes to Kurt and no to the tumor. If you want to say yes to life, you have to say yes to all of it."

"Are you sure? Because I really, really want to say no to this tumor."

"You can try, but it will cause you a lot more suffering. This isn't about whether you'll die or not. We know you're going to die, I'm going to die; everyone dies. This is about how you want to live until you die. Do you want to live full of fear and worry? Or do you want to say yes to life and live full of gratitude and ease?"

"Oh, please. You sound like me when I give the kids a ridiculous choice, 'Do you want to whine and walk to the airport, or do you want to be quiet and let me drive you there?' "

"It's only ridiculous because it is hard. But you forget how strong you are."

I send him back three emojis: the strong arm, the thumbs up, and the praying hands as thank you.

I am back at the hospital. Dr. Liebsch, the radiation specialist, wants detailed images of my head and neck in order to understand my situation better. Dr. Liebsch has silver hair but looks younger than his sixty-some years. He is not very tall and has a soft, round face. He explains complex issues in a thick German accent with a voice just above a whisper as he calmly waves away concerns with long fingers and manicured nails. But looks are deceptive; Dr. Liebsch is tough, strict, and fiercely dedicated to getting the details right. He spends hours crafting a fiberglass mask of my face and neck to hold my head in exactly the same position every time I have images taken. I like his fastidiousness; it is a good quality in someone who is in charge of radiating your skull. But it's his uncompromising side that can make things difficult.

To make sure that the color contrast for the images saturates my brain and not my feet, Dr. Liebsch straps my ankles into leather buckles and suspends me completely upside down on an examining table. I lie there, feeling blood and contrast rush to my head. I feel like I am going to be sick, but I hold my breath and wait.

When he finally turns me right side up, I throw up several times into a biohazard bin. Throwing up is never fun, but throwing up with a neck fusion is a whole new kind of painful. I am having a rare, unexpected, bad reaction to the contrast. It's not dangerous, just annoying.

"You ok?" Dr. Liebsch asks.

I give the thumbs up.

"Good," he says, "Now you must lie on the floor and roll around to mix the contrast up." I wait to see if he is joking, but he only gives me his hand to help me off the table. I slowly lie down on the cold, tile floor. Then I roll back and forth with all the grace of someone in a hospital gown and neck brace who has just thrown up several times. When they say I can stop, I crawl back onto the table and lie flat on my back. Then they press the fiberglass mask tightly over my face and neck to keep me still, before sliding me into the MRI machine for forty-five minutes. The technician hands me a remote control to stop the machine, in case I feel like throwing up again. But Dr. Liebsch, who is focused on getting all of the images he needs, says, "Don't push the button."

When the scan is over, I only throw up once. Then I meet Kurt in the waiting room where he points out that my hospital gown has just one working tie at the neck and the rest is wide open to the world. I wonder what my dance on the tile floor looked like. Meanwhile, the fire alarm is going off in the hospital, so we leave, despite a nurse saying, "It's nothing. It's nothing."

Outside, the fresh air feels cool on my face and I instantly feel better. Until suddenly, I don't. The next thing I know, I am on my hands and knees in the middle of the street, naked except for my useless gown, throwing up, while Kurt tries to wave traffic around me. I keep thinking, this is as tough as childbirth. Then the puke starts coming out my nose and I can't breathe. No, this is way worse than childbirth.

Finally, it is over. We walk back to our car, and pass a hotel on our way. An older bellhop gives me a big smile. I am still in my ridiculous hospital gown and so I am not really in the mood to be seen, but he seems genuinely able to ignore my outfit.

"My name is Thomas. In Jamaica, where I come from, we like to make people happy. May I sing you a song?"

"Uh. Okay," I say, hesitantly.

And right there, on the sidewalk, Thomas sings to me.

"Three little birds
Pitched by my doorstep,
Singin' sweet songs
Of melodies pure and true
Sayin' this is my message to you,
Singin' don't worry 'bout a thing
'Cause every little thing gonna be alright"

I smile for the first time in days because I believe it. Thomas notices the smile.

"See, I make you happy!" he laughs.

"Thank you," I say. And I mean it.

⋇

The phone rings. It is Dr. Liebsch.

"I've looked at your images and spoken to Dr. Al-Mefty. We don't think you need more surgery now. Let's see if radiation can reduce the spot of tumor on your spine," Dr. Liebsch says without emotion.

"Oh, thank you! That is good news. How much radiation? Four weeks?"

"No. Eight weeks. Every day. Starting in a few days."

"Can I do that from home?"

"The kind of radiation you need is only in eight places across the country. There is not a facility in Colorado. I suggest you stay in Boston and have the radiation done here."

Eight more weeks away from home and the kids. I inhale the news. Then I exhale relief that I don't need more surgery now.

I think back to my conversation with Michael. I'm still uncomfortable with the idea of surrender. But maybe the word I can get behind is "trust." I can work on trusting life more. I trust that I can endure discomfort. *Can I trust that life will hold me for eight more weeks?*

18

It's September 21, the fall equinox. Kurt and the kids are home in Colorado. I am still in Boston for thirty-eight radiation treatments. Every day except weekends, for eight weeks, I'll commute to Massachusetts General Hospital from Jamaica Plain. I'm living with Polly and Bob Thomas, a couple who graciously offers me a room in their home. I taught their daughter high school English seven years ago, but never met them before. They are both cancer survivors, so it's nice to be around people who know what it feels like to go through treatments.

The first morning after radiation, I feel fine. The second day, I can't even get out of bed to get myself a glass of water. Today, I celebrate the elegant evenness of the equinox by throwing up all over a neighbor's garden. The nausea is caused by the radiation, but the feeling of being off-balance is caused by my too-high expectations.

Fear shows up uninvited, saying mean-spirited things like: "This is just the beginning and you can't get out of bed; How are you going to make it through thirty-eight treatments? You said you were going to write! Get up!" I am not practicing good self-compassion because I have unreasonable expectations for these eight weeks. I think that since I am not working and the children are taken care of at home, I should balance my time better and be mega-productive. I think, maybe I can even write a book while I am here. I wish I were kidding. I forget that what makes balancing a trick is precisely that it is extraordinary, like the equinox, or like the street performer who steadies himself on a twenty-foot unicycle.

The way American culture emphasizes balance makes me feel like I should figure out how to be more physically, mentally, and spiritually poised every. single. day. Even before, when I wasn't doing radiation treatments, I would get stressed because I worked too much and played too little, or played too much and worked too little, or ate too much and exercised too little, or exercised too much and wrote too little.

What I want to change is not my reality (which is that I barely have enough energy to make it to my radiation appointment each day), but my expectations. This equinox, I lie in bed, nibble on a saltine cracker, and vow to lower my expectations. I trust that a feeling of balance will occur as a rare and wonderful thing.

⁂

Meanwhile, there is nothing on TV except the presidential candidates hurling insults at one another. No wonder I feel nauseated all the time. I feel helpless. I keep thinking, *How are we going to pull through this as a country? We are divided beyond repair.* Again, I am expecting balance instead of this painful push and pull of different worldviews. But my expectations just leave me feeling frustrated and angry. I'm willing to try something new.

On Sunday, Polly and Bob ask if I want to go to church with them.

"No, thanks," I say. I am not a church goer. Besides, I don't want to sit in a room full of strangers. But, I don't feel like watching TV either. And, I'm a little bit curious.

"Give me a minute," I say, and do my best to dress up by wearing boots instead of running shoes. Polly and Bob seem happy that I want to go.

It is not crowded inside the church; people could have had a whole pew to themselves if they wanted. Instead, strangers slide in side by side so that old white women and young black men, gay couples and straight, are sitting next to me, the weird lady in the neck brace, as if we all arrived in the same station wagon. When it is time to turn to our neighbors and say, "Peace be with you," several people reach across the aisle to shake my hand, though they don't know anything about me.

This coming together of very different kinds of people gives me the same feeling of connection that I have had ever since I first received this tumor diagnosis. It reminds me of the old barn-raising approach—that a group can build something much larger together than any one family could do on its own. Total strangers have reached out to us in ways that we could not have imagined. Buddhists are chanting my name in upstate New York and Christians have created prayer circles for me in Australia. Ordinary people, of all different faiths, offer us support. It's generous and kind. Just yesterday, Polly made my bed with clean, warm sheets and Bob brought me a supper of an omelet made with fresh tomatoes and cheese. I didn't even have to get out of bed to eat it.

In church, we stand to sing the hymn "Sanctuary." "With thanksgiving, I'll be a living sanctuary." I look around. The man in front of me is wearing lavender pants and a lavender t-shirt with a giant dragonfly printed on the back. He has a deep, low voice and he is singing at full volume with his whole heart. Next to him, a young woman in a black leather jacket and black jeans has a voice like a melodious flute. I am inspired. I open my mouth to join in. My voice squeaks and groans like a cold set of bagpipes. So I hum along instead. I notice how different everyone's voice is. Together, we all sound pretty good.

19

It's Halloween, my favorite holiday. I am homesick and I miss my kids. They still dress up and go out trick-or-treating. Cole wants to be Santa Claus, and Hazel wants to be "starlight," as in light from the stars. I just want to be there, with them, and not here. Still, I've dressed up as a disco queen to go to my radiation session, just for fun. I walk into the Burr Proton Beam Therapy Center, and the clinical smell of the hospital fills me with dread. I suddenly feel the weight of why I am separated from my family. *What am I doing in this ridiculous costume? How can I make light of something so serious? What is fun about disease?*

Then, Aïsha, age five, Feliz, age three, and Clayton, age two, walk into the waiting room with their shaved heads and a kind of I-own-this-place swagger. We see each other every day for these two months for radiation treatments. They come from all over the world, but they have one thing in common: they have brain tumors, and are doing chemotherapy and radiation at the same time. They endure several energy-sucking, nausea-inducing sessions a day. But they don't weigh down their experiences with worry and premature grief.

Today, Clayton looks invincible in his red cape, and Aïsha looks glamorous in her blue and silver *Frozen* princess dress. Next, Feliz comes running over to me in her bright pink superhero costume. She yanks out her pacifier, and says with a big smile, "I'm Supergirl!"

"Yes you are!" I say, and we flex muscles together for a while.

Then she asks, "What are you?"

"I'm a disco queen," I say matter-of-factly, in my blonde afro wig, black jumper, seventies-style beads that I borrowed from my friend Karen, and disco-ball earrings.

"Is that a dancer?" she asks.

"Yes! Do you remember showing me that the lights around our radiation machine can change colors, from pink to yellow to blue to green, like a dance floor?"

"Oh yeah!" She says, remembering.

"You gave me the idea to be a dance star for Halloween," I say.

"Dance party!" she shouts and pops her pacifier back in her mouth, shaking her hips. We ask the nurses to change the Pandora radio station to ABBA and to put the lights on "disco mode." Then, we dance. I turn to her mother and say, "Feliz is teaching me how to bring joy to my radiation treatments." She laughs, but then says seriously, "Every day, Feliz teaches me how to live with more joy."

※

Only nine days after Halloween, it is the 2016 American presidential election. The country seems anxious, but I feel positive and optimistic. My last radiation treatment is tomorrow. And we will have a woman president.

I wake up early to make it to the hospital before 8:00 a.m. I feel light and excited. Soon I'll be home with my kids. I pick the newspaper up off the front steps, wet from a gentle morning rain.

The Boston Globe headline essentially shouts at me, YOU ARE WRONG. I stand in the rain, smelling the cold air, watching a few oak leaves tumble to the ground. On the pendulum from fear to trust, I swing all the way back to fear, and am stuck there as anxious thoughts ring in my ears. *We are not safe. We are divided. If I am wrong about the election, am I wrong about my health, too? Maybe the surgeries and the radiation won't work.*

At the hospital, Clayton, Aïsha, and Feliz are not there. The receptionist tells me that the radiation machine is broken. There won't be any treatments today. "Go home," the receptionist says.

"I wish I could," I feel like telling her. Today, I thought I was going to put the tumor behind me. Today, I thought we would have a woman president. Today, I thought I would be able to go home with my family. But I need one more treatment. It's not over yet.

I call Kurt while sitting on a bench in the Boston Public Garden. I cry a little to him on the phone and say, "The radiation machine is broken. And our country is divided. I have to come back and do more radiation. What if they don't fix the machine? What if we can't fix the country?"

"Can we be grateful that you only have one more treatment left, before rushing to thoughts of a dark future?" Kurt responds, teasing me a little.

Can I feel grateful now? I don't know. It feels awkward, like kneeling to pray on a hard floor. It also feels creaky, like the sound of a screen door opening. Worrying about the future is my stupid, secret superpower. The only thing that comes to me is, "I am thankful that I am not pregnant right now."

I'm learning that giving thanks is both a refuge and a protector. I picture it like a Hindu goddess with a Canadian-girl twist; she sits in lotus position and has four arms, but she wears a red coat like a Mountie. One of her hands carries a sword to fight off dark thoughts. One carries a shield as protection from maladies. One holds a flower and points to the earth as a safe shelter, and the last one is empty, open to the unknown.

Then I remember a trick my therapist taught me. "When gratitude is difficult to find in the present, make up a scene in the future that makes you feel thankful. Then marinate in that feeling." On the bench in the garden, watching strangers rush past me in coats and scarves, I try it.

I lob myself into a make-believe future like winter's first snowball and I dream up something ridiculous and wonderful. I imagine that I am an old, healthy woman full of stories and soft wrinkles, sitting on a sunny porch overlooking the ocean. I am holding Cole's firstborn child and teaching her the Latin names of birds like *Fregata magnificens*. Family and friends swing open our cabin's screen door, kiss me and the baby, and run along a tropical trail to a wide, sandy beach with left-breaking, blue-green waves. A scratchy radio plays in the background. Our president announces that she has made a peace accord with North Korea, similar to the one she made with Afghanistan years earlier. I hold Cole's precious baby in my arms. She smells like fresh beginnings and I breathe her in deeply as I walk slowly down to the beach in my frilly, old-lady, bathing suit.

Fear, the know-it-all professor, says that my vision is "Cute, but not very realistic." I ignore her and I let the dream wash over me like a warm ocean wave. For a moment, I let myself bathe in deep contentment.

20

A few days later, the radiation machine is fixed. Kurt and the kids arrive in Boston to bring me home. We arrive at my last treatment with presents and cake for Aïsha, Clayton, and Feliz. In turn, they hug our kids tight like family. When I say goodbye to Feliz, I get teary, because I may never see her again. "The best is yet to come," I say to her. And she says it right back to me. It's what we say after each treatment, when parting. It feels better than saying goodbye.

Next, I write an email to our friends saying, "We did it! Ring a bell (cow, bike, door) to celebrate your positivity, the end of radiation treatments, and healing." A friend texts me from New York to say that her power is out; she can't ring her doorbell in solidarity with me. Instead, she says, "I'm banging on every pot and pan I can find to celebrate. Can you hear me?"

Home in Colorado, we invite our families to join us for Thanksgiving dinner. It's a large, eclectic group. Our family includes Republicans and Democrats, gay and straight people, gun lovers and anti-gun activists. I don't really know where to seat people. I move name plates around, anxiously. Then everyone arrives, and we light candles on the table, each one symbolic of someone or something we are grateful for in our lives.

We light candles for Aïsha, Clayton, and Feliz. The grandparents light candles for their grandchildren. My in-laws light candles for their parents. The activists light candles for community organizers. Our kids light candles for pointe shoes and skateboards. My mom lights a candle for Roger Federer, the tennis great. When we're done, there are hundreds of candles lit on every free space on the table. Gratitude is bonding. We are not the same. But we come together in solidarity when we focus on what we appreciate. Our home smells of roast turkey, rich gravy, and candle wax. The room is full of light. We raise our glasses in thanksgiving, and celebrate.

≈≈≈

Before I went into surgery, I asked myself, *If you come out of this unscathed, with a full life ahead of you, How are you going to live? Will you do anything differently?*

When death had me in her clutches, it was easy to know how to live:

Slow down.

Do less.

Write more.

And let joy lead.

But now that I'm home, without a job, and with kids to care for, the wisdom I learned feels remote and a little reckless. I see myself slipping back into old patterns, like worrying about where to seat people for Thanksgiving dinner. *Can I really integrate what I've learned into daily life?* I am determined to try. *What does choosing brave over perfect look like now?*

Tell the Truth

With the diagnosis, I worried, When will I lose my voice? But the real question became, When did I let it go? We unapologetically express ourselves when we are really young. Then we start lying. We lie to hide our struggles or we lie to please others. We lie when we pretend to be someone we are not. We lie when w curate our lives on social media. Gradually, by constantly lying, or at least not telling our inner truth, we lose touch with who we are. Have you ever held back in a discussion, not saying what you strongly felt? If you share that thing with just one person, even now, you'll feel better. You'll feel more *you*.

To reclaim our voices, we need to tell the truth:

- *Use "no" as your samurai sword*. Say no to what you think you *should* do. Make room for what you *love* to do. Walk out of that movie. Decline that party invitation. Step down from that committee. Practice making decisions from a place of inner truth, not outer expectation.

- *Say less, listen more*. Do you talk to understand, or to prove that you are right, or to influence the outcome? Imagine that tomorrow you have your annual review at work, or that you need to talk with your teenager about college applications. Picture yourself in that conversation. What do you usually say in similar moments? Now, picture yourself being as succinct as possible, saying only what truly matters to these people you value. What would you say now? Next, listen. Your truest words will come from listening and understanding.

- *Create a morning routine* in which the first eleven minutes of your day are quiet, slow, and solitary. Eleven minutes because it is doable daily. Write in your journal. Slice oranges. Don't speak, check your phone, or read the headlines. If you have a kid, don't make their lunch. If you always run or workout with other people, meet them somewhere eleven minutes from your house so the first minutes are yours to feel what you feel in silence. Begin each day by grounding yourself in you before responding to others.

- *See yourself as part of something larger.* Every voice matters. Even the kid in the back who isn't singing but is stomping his foot to the beat, belongs in the choir. Too often we get caught up thinking that we have nothing special to offer. *I don't have anything to say.* Take the pressure off of your shoulders, and imagine that something wants to be said *through* you. I believe in a kind of stone soup philosophy; none of us knows what we have until we put it all together. I'll bring an onion, if you bring a carrot, and someone else brings salted water. Collectively, we'll make a damn good soup.

- *If you can't say it, try writing it.* When it comes time to express how we truly feel, our fear of rejection is strong. I am thinking about big things like forgiving your parents, apologizing to someone, or talking about sex with your teenager. These are too important to skip. Write down what is in your heart and read what you have written instead.

- *Your voice is an instrument.* Get curious about it. Take singing lessons. It doesn't matter if you are tone-deaf or have zero ambitions to be Beyoncé. Besides being fun, you'll discover how to use this powerful tool to create a life you love.

PART IV

METAMORPHOSIS

21

One morning in December, I wake up full of rage. I angry-clean the coffee grounds in the sink. (Angry-clean: verb. To make loud, banging noises and swear under your breath while scrubbing or vacuuming or generally tidying up.)

I yell at our son, "Get out of the bathroom! I need to get in!" Then I scream at our daughter for not moving faster to get ready for school. "Hurry up! You're going to make us all late!" Next I huff and puff around my husband during breakfast, hollering, "Put your phone down and help me!" He raises an eyebrow, puts his phone down, and walks out of the room. On the kitchen table, his screen is still illuminated. I see that he is working on paying my medical bills.

I have no idea what to do with all this rage. I pour myself a strong cup of green tea. Like a good girl, I wash my morning vitamins down with the tea. My throat burns. Since the surgeries, my throat often hurts because the tumor damaged some of the muscles and nerves in that area. But this feeling is different; it feels tight, as if I am afraid of what words might come out if I open my mouth.

Where is all this emotion coming from? Maybe my anger this morning is because I listened to the news until late last night. The news makes me feel powerless against the mounting ways that the world is unjust and unsafe. Maybe it's more personal than that. Before, I believed that if I followed the rules and was good in all the ways that a girl is "supposed" to be good, the world would reward me with kindness and freedom. But instead I was handed an incurable, terminal illness.

Next, I do what I have always done when I feel like I'm going to explode. I walk to the front door and grab my running shoes. In the past, when I felt angry, sad, or scared, I numbed myself by running for hours or making myself so busy that I didn't have time to feel the pain of dark emotions. I wanted to get as far away as possible from uncomfortable feelings like anger. I didn't realize that I was just storing the rage inside.

"Where are you going?" Kurt asks.

"For a slow jog. I need to get out of here."

"You can't run, remember? It's not safe." Kurt says.

His words sting like rocks to the flesh. And not only because they remind me that I am broken and fragile. They trigger something deep inside me. I've heard that phrase my whole life. It's not safe to walk at night. It's not safe to wear that. It's not safe to go there. It's not safe to travel by yourself. It's not safe to drive those roads. It's not safe to accept a drink from someone. It's not safe to be alone, ever. Why not? Shouldn't it be just as safe for me as it is for you? I want to scream.

I slam my shoes down on the floor. Then I walk past Kurt and the kids; the fire behind my throat feels hotter and I can't ignore it anymore. I need water. I'm in the kitchen. Then suddenly, my legs feel weak and buckle under me. I throw up into the trash can. The vomit is green from all those multivitamins and green tea I took earlier. I don't feel hot or clammy or cramped. There is nothing wrong with me, except that I took some strong pills on an empty stomach. But is it a coincidence that I threw up after feeling all that rage?

I don't think so. I have spent my whole life being the good girl. Good girls don't express rage. It's no wonder that I have no idea what to do with the anger that consumes me sometimes. I will not stay quiet. I want to speak up for what matters to me. But if I don't process and express the rage I feel in a healthy way, I will throw up all over the people closest to me.

Since running is no longer an option, I turn to writing. I take off my sneakers and head downstairs to the guest room where I've set up an old table as a desk. I pick up my journal. My hand shakes, but I can't stop scribbling angry words on the page. I write:

Sometimes there is a rage inside me that is not mine, but ours. Rage for the tumor stripping me of a strong voice. Rage for generations of voiceless and silenced people. Rage for living in fear of what my future and my children's future holds. Rage for those who live in fear because of their gender, their class, or the color of their skin. Rage for those who are raped and for those who are abused. Rage for the poverty that too many are born into. Rage for the privilege that I was born into. Rage for the feeling of helplessness. Rage that I am not angrier, not doing more.

I feel strangely better writing about what makes me mad. My mind wanders to an exchange yesterday afternoon on the playground. I'm there to pick up my daughter from school. Hazel is hanging from the top bar of the swing set, about fifteen feet off the ground.

A man in a dark coat approaches. I don't recognize him.

He asks me, "Is that your daughter up there?"

"Yes," I say, proudly.

"It's not safe," the man says, and shakes his head. "Tell her to come down."

"Oh, of course," I say without thinking. I feel ashamed. *I should have made her come down sooner.* This man must know more than I do about the dangers involved. *I didn't protect her. I am a bad mom.* But then I look at my daughter and remember how strong she is. I feel suddenly defiant; I don't ask her to come down.

"Thank you," I say to the man. "But she'll be alright up there."

He frowns. I stand my ground. I'm tired of hearing people tell me, "It's not safe."

I am tired of the reality that it is not safe anywhere, as the news reports and documentaries pile up with horrifying stories, sounding that same note over and over to women: "It's not safe, it's not safe, it's not safe." I am especially tired of hearing myself tell my daughter, "It's not safe." Yesterday, I remember saying that phrase to her at least four times. *It's not safe to run up the slide, to jump off that boulder, to climb on the swing set, to talk to strangers.* There is a need to be alert to the dangerous forces out there. But there is also a need to stop marinating my daughter in fear. I want her to discover that she is strong, she is capable, and that she can swing from the high bar as much as she wants.

It makes me think about my own relationship with the world. As I write in my journal, I realize something important. My perfectionism comes from a feeling that the world is not safe. I am motivated by fear. *It's not safe to fail. It's not safe to be average. It's not safe to begin before I'm completely ready. It's not safe to believe that all will be well. It's not safe to count on responding positively when bad things happen.*

Typically, I caution and warn my daughter with stories and worst-case scenarios in an effort to protect her. The problem is she takes on my fears and insecurities like armor. Unfortunately, they don't protect my daughter; they only shield the world from her unique awesomeness. *How can I raise her to be brave if I am afraid of being anything less than perfect?*

The trick, I'm realizing, is not to run from anger or fear, but to feel them, deeply. Before, I thought I was brave because I pushed past pain. But bravery is facing fear, being vulnerable, and sitting in discomfort with anger.

Once Kurt leaves for work and the kids go to school, I settle into the blue chair in the corner of the room with my journal. I close my eyes. What does rage feel like in my body? I notice a tightness in my throat, like I am choking, and a hardness in my stomach. I wonder, *Am I going to be sick again? Or is that just what anger feels like?* As I write about what I am feeling, my throat softens. Then I let out a long, painful wail. It is deep, and low, and shakes my whole body. I catch my breath, and do it again. And again. I am grateful that no one is in the house to hear me. *Why? Shouldn't they hear this? This is what it means to be a woman. This is what it means to be human. We feel pain.*

Expressing how I feel might be the most radical thing I can do to heal. I give myself permission to feel the pain, and the fiery thoughts I had minutes ago loosen their grip. My stomach relaxes. Instead of rushing around the house, spreading anxiety with my misdirected tirades, I feel calm. I feel grounded enough to get up and do normal things, like brush my teeth.

Then I go to the grocery store. I notice my neighbor in the produce section, choosing avocados from an overflowing pile. I smile at her, and she looks at me strangely. I immediately jump to the first five things I must have done wrong. *Did I not respond to an email? Or send her a thank you card? Did I forget her birthday? Is she embarrassed that I'm wearing floral Hawaiian pajamas to the store? What's wrong with me?*

Turns out, my neighbor didn't even notice my pajamas. And I didn't forget her birthday. She forgot her glasses at home. She wasn't judging me or looking at me strangely. She was just squinting because she couldn't see.

There's nothing wrong with me; it's just that I have this inner critic who takes his job really seriously. He is Fear's inventive cousin, who has me imagining that everyone is mad at me, all the time. *Your neighbor thinks you are a lousy friend. Kurt is angry that you snapped at him this morning and didn't help with dinner last night. The kids are mad that you don't play with them enough. No one likes it when you wear pajamas to the store.*

Back home, I head straight for the blue chair. *Why do I think people are mad at me all the time?* What comes to me is this: The tumor grew mainly on the medulla oblongata, the part of the brain that some refer to as the fight-or-flight center. I am ready at any moment to fight or run for my safety.

I am afraid that I am not enough as I am. I'm afraid I'm letting my parents down, my kids down, my husband down, and my friends down, all the time. I fill my days with busywork so that I can point to what I've done that day and say, *See? I'm chipping in. I'm worthy. Will you love me now? Please don't be mad at me.*

Maybe my anger and my perception of others' anger are linked to not feeling safe. Some part of me must believe I am not safe. It's not safe to live in this world as I am. It's not safe to be one-hundred-percent me.

I notice an old photograph that is taped to the base of the lamp on my desk. It's me at two years old on the red sand of a beach on Prince Edward Island, near my grandmother's home. I am wearing a white and pink jumper that is soaked through from an encounter with ocean waves. *Of course you are enough,* I say to the innocent girl in the picture. *You are loved. You belong here. You are safe.* Suddenly, I have a desire to write a letter to that little girl.

I pick up my pen. *Honey, we're going to burn off some of that insecurity right now.*

> Dear Little Susie,
>
> Baby girl, you can't live like this, full of fear and doubt. I see you at two years old, with a look of joyful surprise on your face, full of wonder. But by eight years old, you think you are too loud, too needy, and too sensitive to be loved. You wonder, *Why can't I do the right thing and not mess up?* You can't forget the time that you were supposed to set the table for dinner. You wanted it to be special,

so you found candles and lit them. You didn't know they would drip and burn your grandmother's crocheted tablecloth. You just wanted to be helpful, but you are always so clumsy.

And then you notice that you get a lot of attention when you achieve. Dad hugs you tight when you show him your perfect score on your spelling test. Mom tells her friends about the 800-meter race you won at the track meet. So achieving seems like an answer. If you just keep bringing home perfect scores and winning races, then you'll be adding value to the family and to the world. Then you'll be loved. Then you'll be safe.

I'm here to tell you, as your older, wiser self, you are safe right now. You are loved exactly as you are: emotional, energetic, willful you. It doesn't matter if you fail a spelling test or fifty spelling tests, you're safe. You will not be left behind or alone.

I'm sorry that I've been so busy achieving in order to earn love that I haven't been here for you. I'm here now. And I'm never going to leave you. You're enough. It is safe to be one-hundred-percent you are, exactly as you are.

I get it. There were times when you did not feel like the world was a safe place. After all, your parents split up and your father moved out. And you didn't know anyone who just had one parent at home. Maybe, you thought, if you were less messy, loud, and chaotic, he'd come back. Maybe if you worked harder, ran faster, did more, no one would leave you alone again.

I will never leave you. I want to hold you in my arms and have you breathe in all this love. You are a perfect human being, growing exactly as you should grow. To be human means to be a contradictory, confusing creature. You are clumsy and graceful. You are selfish and thoughtful. You have a bad temper and you are calm. You are fragile and you are strong. This is who you are. No matter how you show up, you deserve to be here. You belong here.

Wait. There's more. You never quite got how exceptional you really are. It's time for you to believe it and step into your infinite power.

Love,
Susie

I put my pen down. Tears are falling down my face. Whether I am raging at the world or raging at myself, it's all feels violent. *I am done with violence.* I want to show up as beautifully flawed and totally in love with the world, no matter how messy and unsafe it can be.

22

A few weeks later, I lie in bed, unable to sleep. I feel like I have forgotten everything I learned about making friends with myself and the world. I slide into that old habit of spinning with anxious thoughts. I blame it on the wind.

The wind is kicking up everything. It's knocking over trash cans and basketball hoops in driveways. Tree branches snap to the ground, blocking sidewalks. A blue patio umbrella sails over the road and lands like a javelin in the sewer grate.

The wind is kicking up my anxious energy. Fear wants me to be awake, and afraid. She whispers in my ear, "What if the old cottonwood falls on the house? What if the windows break in the children's room? What if it starts to rain, we lose power, and then have massive flooding?"

I get up to crank the bathroom window closed and the wind grabs the frame. "Stop! Stop! Stop!" I yell at the wind and use all my strength to resist its pull. I see my face in the mirror and notice how dark and small my eyes are above my tense lips. I am not just resisting the wind. I am fighting everything.

When I can't control the weather, or my health, or what the president says, or how my husband behaves, I can't sleep. I can't feel at peace. I want things to be different than they are. I want them to be how *I* think they should be. *The wind should stop. The president should listen more. My husband should understand me better. Life should be less painful.* Where do those thoughts get me? I'm sleep-deprived and angry. I know that the outside events are not the problem. My desire to control what happens in the world is the problem. But I'm finding it difficult to live knowing that. *Can I accept myself and things as they are, and move forward anyway?*

I step into the wind. I put on my warmest jacket and pull the hood tight around my face. I walk ten blocks to Raj yoga studio to sign up for a forty-day meditation course called "Journey to the Self." I want to do this to manage my thoughts. I want more calm and clarity, and less anger and anxiety.

The yoga studio is in a commercial building next to an auto shop, a marijuana dispensary, and a dingy western bar. But inside the studio, everything is white and luminescent. I sit on a folded blanket near the back of the room and look around. There are a dozen women and two men, all wearing white flowing pants. I am in black sweats. *They look like angels. I look like I'm ready to box. I don't belong here.* Above, I can hear the wind lifting the edge of the metal roof and rattling it. I feel like the wind is lifting my bones and rattling them, too.

Just then, Sukhraj, the teacher, reminds us, "If you are here, it means you agree to meditate for forty continuous days. It also means you choose to give up sugar, alcohol, caffeine, and meat for forty days." *That seems a little excessive. No coffee? No beer? Or ice cream? For forty days?* But I am ready to do something drastic.

Sukhraj hands each of us a small notebook and says, "Take five minutes. Write down the answer to this question: *What do you want out of this experience?*" I imagine that the flowing-white-pants people are writing noble, peaceful aspirations such as, "To spread peace and goodness in the world." I can't think of anything inspiring. I am ready to get up and leave. Just then the wind hisses and screeches like a train roaring into the yoga studio.

The wind kicks up my courage. I write, "I want to stop fighting the world and find joy. I want to sleep more and spin in my thoughts less.

I want to make friends with the fact that I am not in control of the weather, my health, or the outcome of a recent presidential election."

Sukhraj then asks us to sit up straight, close our eyes, and inhale and exhale through our nose. I am immediately uncomfortable. My back aches and my right knee sends pain signals to my brain. I uncross and recross my legs. I want to be serene, but I am restless and afraid. I'm nervous because I've tried to meditate before. But it doesn't work. My mind wanders and I make endless to-do lists. I never seem to get back to my breath.

This time is no different. My thoughts jump from one escape plan to the next. *I should go. I think I left the stove on at home. And I'm pretty sure the kids have a dentist appointment right now that we're missing. I should check. I'll just make a quick call and come right back.* Then my thoughts turn dark. *I don't want to be here. I don't like these people. I shouldn't have spent the money.* I yell at my thoughts, *Get lost!* but they don't listen. My mind feels like a bouncy castle and my thoughts are toddlers, high on cake.

The wind shakes the windows and slams the yoga room door shut. Sukhraj says, "Our goal is to find steadiness inside and be calm when our thoughts and the wind are whipping around."

It is suddenly months earlier, and I am reliving being alone in the darkness, facing my diagnosis. That is when I have the terrifying thought, *I will die young and without a voice.* I believe it so fully that I go crazy with pain and grief. But then I notice that the tumor itself isn't painful; I can't even feel it in my skull. The tumor isn't causing my suffering, my thoughts are.

Somehow I understand that I am not my thoughts. I am the one hearing them, that's all. This makes me laugh out loud with joy. I can't control what is happening to me physically, but I can control how it affects me. I realize I have a choice. I can choose to believe my thoughts or not. I feel light and absolutely free. I know how I want to face my circumstances and I write my homemade mantra down: "I choose joy over fear and brave over perfect."

But ever since I've been home, after the surgeries, and back into the routine of regular life, Fear keeps cozying up with me and my fiery insides. "Your mantra is cute. But you can't choose joy, just like that. Who do you think you are?" I keep trying to push Fear away to choose joy. But Fear keeps coming back, while joy seems to have left and gone to the beach.

After my first week of meditating in the yoga studio, I call my friend Christine, who is a life coach, to tell her that my mantra is no longer working. She laughs, "It works. Look at how far you've come. You're writing now and sharing your writing! But you can't make fearful thoughts go away. You can only question them. Have you heard of Byron Katie? Go buy one of her books."

I go to the Boulder Bookstore, one of my favorite places in town, and buy *Loving What Is*. Then I sit down on the floor, upstairs in the "personal growth" section, and study Byron Katie's process. "Suffering is optional," says Katie. "It's not the problem that causes us suffering; it's our thinking about the problem." Katie became terribly depressed in her forties. Then one morning, after hitting rock bottom, she woke up full of joy. Through a process of inner questioning, she realized that all her old thoughts were untrue and she didn't need to believe them anymore.

As I read her story, I slap the pages with excitement, *That's what I experienced too! I'm not crazy. It's possible!* A tall man browsing the Zen meditation books gives me a frown, then walks to the other side of the room. I ignore his scowl and get back to my reading. Katie developed "The Work," a series of questions to give herself and others the freedom she felt that morning. A light bulb goes on inside me. I thought that once I had that experience of not believing all my thoughts, I'd never have problems again. I thought it was a one-time-fixes-all kind of insight. But Katie emphasizes that it's a practice.

On day seven of my forty-day meditation, I try out Byron Katie's questions. I sit on my folded blanket, still at the back of the room but more at home than before. I playfully experiment with each thought that arises. *The wind should stop.* "Is that absolutely true?" I ask. I hold the thought up to the light and look at it from all sides. As Katie teaches, I turn it around to see if a different thought feels just as true. *The wind should not stop. The wind is doing exactly what it's supposed to be doing.* That feels more true to reality.

I keep going with each thought that is making me suffer. *The president should listen more.* That's true! I holler in my mind. But I try out another idea that causes me to suffer less. *I can speak up more.*

Another thought pops into my mind. *My husband should understand me better.* I want him to know how I am feeling without having to tell him. But I flip the thought anyway. *I want to understand me better.* Yes. I feel that one soften my throat. How can I expect him to do all the understanding when most of the time I have no idea what I am feeling?

Finally, I look at the thought, *Life should be less painful.* This one feels true. I believe it. There's too much violence and death, and I still have an incurable, terminal disease. *How can I possibly turn this thought around?*

Then I remember something Byron Katie wrote, "Trying to let go of a painful thought never works. Instead, once we question it, the thought lets go of *us.*" I now know my mistake. I have been trying to push my anxious ruminations away instead of sitting with them. But when I try to force them away, Fear's voice gets stronger, louder, and more critical. I take a deep breath.

I see the thought, *Life should be less painful,* on my imaginary blackboard.
I want to erase it. But instead I look at it with curiosity. Really? What
is causing me more pain? Life or my thoughts? I play with the order
of the words. *Life should be less painful* becomes *My thinking could be less
painful.* That resonates. I have enough real physical pain to deal with;
I don't need to make it worse with my thinking. But it's also not saying
I *must* do something to change my thoughts; it's just pointing out that
there is possibility and light here. I exhale. The tight boulder in my
stomach has shrunk to a smooth river stone. My chest feels open and
expansive, buzzing with rebellious pleasure.

My mantra isn't broken. I just need practice. I still have a choice.
Choosing joy over fear isn't about destroying fear. It's about calibrating
my thinking. With a little investigation and courage, I can shift the
equation from being driven by fear to being led by joy.

Then I notice something important. My desire to control how
life should be is another form of perfectionism. When I aim my
perfectionism at myself, it's about not being good enough. Christine is
right; I am making good progress here. Most days I think I am cured
of my perfectionism. I procrastinate less and take more risks. I don't
need to please others as much anymore. I write and post my work
publicly. I've gone from believing that my writing is not worthy of an
audience to thinking, *Oh well. It is good enough.*

But when I turn my gaze outward, my perfectionism is about everyone
and everything else not being good enough. It's all about control. I
have to accept that I am not in charge. And that makes the world too
uncertain for my taste. My taste is to hold the steering wheel, the paper
map, *and* the GPS on life's winding road.

*Can I make friends with a world that is dangerous and out of my control? Can I
accept that life is uncertain, and maybe not what I expected or wanted? Can I admit
that I'm sad and angry about not being in charge?*

I know I haven't fully recovered from perfectionism. As Christine says, "Perfectionism is a little like an addiction, and recovery from it is a little like sobriety. You take it one day at a time."

Inside me, there is a tender transformation happening: away from needing to be in control and toward acceptance and trust. But I expected the change to feel more solid and complete. Like one day, I'm a caterpillar; the next, a butterfly. Instead I still feel like the unformed, green goop inside the cocoon. So I'm learning to celebrate small-but-significant changes, like doing less each day, and being able to say no to invitations that feel like obligations.

The other night, a friend calls to ask if I am coming to their Super Bowl party, even though it is a month away. This friend is family. We have gone to their Super Bowl party every year since we moved to Colorado. But as she is talking and wondering who will perform at the halftime show, I listen to my inner voice. I am surprised by what I really want to say.

"So, do you want to bring chips and guacamole again?" she asks.

"No."

"Ok. Do you want to bring something else?" she pivots, undeterred. I take a deep breath.

"I'm not coming. I love *you*. But I *hate* football. And Sundays are my best writing days."

I wait for the phone to go dead. I wait for her to ask me to take her name off the kids' emergency contact list. I wait for her to point out all the things she has done for me that she didn't want to do. But none of that happens. Her response catches me off guard.

"Good for you! How about a walk next week, instead?" she says, and she doesn't sound hurt or offended. I am giddy. I said no and the only thing that happened was I received a better invitation. I know that this is a small thing, but it feels revolutionary. I remember the euphoria I felt when I walked out of a movie. Learning that it's okay to say no feels like discovering, as a child, that I can float. The water holds. I'm not going to drown.

Each invitation becomes an opportunity to listen to what I really want to do, and not to what I think is expected of me. My neighbor asks if I want to be in her book club. I say, "No, not this time. Sweet of you to ask!" A former colleague asks if I want to join a networking group. I say, "No, thanks!" It turns out that saying no is a great way to find my voice. Every time I say no, I feel defiant in the best possible way. I chase approval and safety from others less. And I feel the tension around my throat release more.

When I say how I feel all day long, there is no trace of resentment in my voice when I come home at night. I am relaxed and not as restless. The kids pick up on my energy. They pile on the couch next to me. They talk over one another as they tell stories of our last camping trip, of eating s'mores and using pine sap like glue to make fairy houses. I scratch their backs and listen. Even in this quiet place, where I don't say a thing, my voice feels true.

These days, I am also a moveable nap. I nap on the couch, in front of a friend's fireplace, or on the floor, drooling on the rug. At first, it frustrates me that, since the surgeries, I can't make it through a day without lying down. Now I think about my naps differently.

In September, I am asleep more than awake and I (mostly) accept that it is part of the healing process. But by October, naps make me feel fragile and old. In November, I call myself weak. One doctor reassures me that short naps, between ten and thirty minutes, do more for lessening anxiety and improving focus than caffeine or even adding an hour of sleep at night.

The feeling that I shouldn't lie down comes from the same shame that I feel if I am not producing something or fixing something. To do nothing feels wrong. But the brave thing for me to do is to nap. There is deep beauty to just being. After a nap, I am more present with the people I love. I am also more positive. I am at least better able to deal with drama.

Now I nap at least once a day. I just napped in the middle of writing this chapter. I love that feeling right before I fall asleep, when I tug a blanket over my shoulders and sink into silence, knowing that soon I will be rested. I focus on that good feeling and ignore the one that says I am not doing enough. By doing less, I feel seen. I feel heard. And the funny thing is, I am the one who is finally seeing, and finally listening, to myself.

I'm discovering that when I say no to things I think I have to do, I make room for things I love to do. I'm writing more now. Before, I worried about getting the words right on the page. Now, I don't care if I am getting them right; I just want to get them down. The way I think about it is this: I didn't grow up wanting to know the perfect stories from perfect people. I wanted to know my mom's stories, and both my grandmothers' stories. I wanted their tales of real struggle and real beauty. But they didn't think they were good enough to write them down. I think it's a mistake to believe we need to be writers with a capital W to put down our stories on paper. I think we should all write as if it's our last chance to be alive and reflect on it. Because it is.

⁓⁓

By day twenty-one, I find it easier to sit still and meditate. The technique Sukhraj has us doing works for me. She puts on beautiful music, then has us cross our arms at the wrists, touch our thumbs to each forefinger, stare at the tip of our nose, and repeat the syllables of a simple mantra. It's enough of a tap-your-head, rub-your-belly, experience that my mind doesn't run away as quickly. I can stay in the moment longer.

After class, my friend Teresa and I walk partway up Mt. Sanitas. It's the small mountain just west of my house whose name literally translates to Mt. Health. Teresa and I used to come here all the time. When I was training for ultramarathons, we divided the mountain trail into chapters, as if it were a book. I used to be able to run to the summit of the mountain, all six chapters, in fewer than twenty-one minutes. Today I only make it to chapter two, and it takes me fifteen minutes. I tell Teresa to go on without me. I need to turn around. I'm tired and my neck fusion hurts.

Then I notice a woman in a blue sweatshirt with Middlebury written in white block letters on the front. Teresa and I both went to Middlebury College. This woman is much younger than us, and she is running fast toward us on the path where I am slowly walking. Teresa waves excitedly, with maybe a little too much enthusiasm, and not enough explanation. The woman wears a confused smile, and keeps running. I want to shout, *Can't you run on another trail? You're breaking my heart!* I feel a mix of envy and grief. I too want to feel that runner's high. I too want to be training for something exciting. I'd like to at least jog a 5K fun run with my kids. But I can't anymore. My spine is fused from my skull to my shoulders. It is held together with metal rods and screws. Running could loosen that hardware, or break it.

I think about Middlebury—about the days when I was captain of the track team and ended up on the wall of fame in the athletic field house. And I think about how I am a walker now. I feel tremendously small and slow and sad. I have to admit to myself that I thought my ability to run fast over thirty miles, no sweat, was proof that I was different, and special. But now, I wonder, *How am I extraordinary if I can't run?*

I look up and notice the morning light hitting the rocks and a red-tailed hawk flying overhead. I remember that I'm out here because I love being outside, surrounded by nature and friends, not because I want to summit the mountain in twenty minutes. I realize I have the thought backwards. It's not about the world celebrating me. It's about me celebrating the world. The question isn't, *How am I extraordinary if I can't run?*

The real question is, *How is the world extraordinary?*

It feels good to take the pressure off my shoulders. I don't have to be exceptional to belong here on Earth. I am here. Therefore, I belong here. I keep walking, and I see shades of green I've never noticed before on the hillside. And I like seeing those colors. I suddenly don't mind walking instead of running. I am grateful for all that I notice, moving at this pace in the world, beyond fear.

On day twenty-eight, Sukhraj says, "When you are not afraid to face life as it is, your frustration relaxes. You can step into the wind and transform your negativity into something good and positive."

She gives us time to write in our notebooks. I write, "The wind is unsettling, yes. So is the world. So is life. So is the unknown. Deeply, deeply unsettling. I lost something important to me in running. But I'm learning to slow down. Now I notice the hummingbird shaking the rain off its wings. I smell the butterscotch scent in a ponderosa pine tree. I am finding unexpected joys everywhere."

On day thirty-five, I step into the wind. I might not be able to run, but I can dance. Sort of. Kurt and I take our first ballroom dance class. It's something I have wanted to do forever, but I dismissed the idea as ridiculous. I was also convinced that Kurt would never want to go. He's more of a hunting and fishing kind of guy. So I never asked, until last week. I bring it up after dinner one night, and Kurt surprises me by saying, "That sounds fun."

The Arthur Murray dance studio is in a run-down mall on the edge of town. The room is small and dark, except for one wall that is all mirrors and a single strand of Christmas lights dangling across the top. The wooden floors are roughed up from people dancing in high heels. I am wearing running shoes.

Our instructor, Isaac, greets us in a brown suit and gold tie. He says, "We're going to do the cha cha. But don't worry, you can rumba to any cha cha."

"Somebody pinch me!" says Kurt, just to me, feigning enthusiasm. I have no idea how to do either dance. I feel my desire to impress Isaac creep into the room. I want to dazzle him with my ability to learn the "boom chica chica" rhythm faster than any student he has ever had before. I speed up the steps, and start telling Kurt where to put his feet. Then I catch myself, and laugh.

This is not a contest or a race; it is a dance. I slow down, look into Kurt's eyes, and listen to the music. It feels amazing to be held, to look at him, to touch hands, to move across the floor without caring where I put my feet next. We cannot stop smiling. This is what it feels like to let joy lead.

"You two have a lot of potential," says Isaac. "I think you're almost ready to learn the Magic Right Turn."

"Somebody pinch me!" I say to Kurt, and crack up.

The forty days of my meditation journey are almost up. I notice that I have slipped and had coffee, sugar, bacon, and beer a few times, but

I haven't missed a day of meditating. I also haven't yelled at my kids once this month. Every day, I wake up in the dark to light a single candle and meditate for at least eleven minutes. I cherish the quiet moment to myself. And when I'm still, I can hear joy's whimsical voice deep inside, guiding me.

Kurt and I continue to go to dance classes. We laugh a lot together. The wind still roars and rages sometimes, but it doesn't bother me as much. Lately, the most delicious thing has been happening. At night, I crawl in bed, I close my eyes, and I sleep. I don't wake with anxious thoughts. I sleep soundly, deeply, like someone who has just been born.

23

I wake up eight hours later with a single idea: "I want to find a new voice coach." I email my friend Dr. Beth Osnes, a theater professor at the University of Colorado, who puts me in touch with Gillian, an opera singer.

I have my first lesson on a rainy Friday in December. In her twenties, Gillian lost her voice and, temporarily, her career. "I learned a lot from my opera training, but I learned more from having to find my voice again," Gillian tells me. We sit in her small home office in Boulder. There isn't much in the office except for a keyboard and a giant scratching post. Her cat ignores the scratching post. It sits at my feet, rubbing itself on my boots.

"I am hoping you can help me speak without pain or effort," I tell Gillian.

"What's the problem?"

"I have to force air out to make sounds that people can hear. By the end of a five-minute conversation, I'm exhausted."

"Oh honey, I'm going to have you singing in no time," she responds.

"No, no, I don't sing. I'm here to learn to talk," I correct her.

"Can you do this?" she ignores me, and lip trills like a baby blowing a raspberry.

I laugh and do my best lip trill, which sounds like a very weak, unripe raspberry.

"Now, lip trill 'We Three Kings' with me," she says and moves to the keyboard.

I have no idea what this has to do with speaking clearly. But I am a little bit scared of her and I do what she says. The cat moves on to rub its back on Gillian's leg.

I lip-trill "we" perfectly, but "three kings" comes out sounding like a boat motor sputtering from lack of fuel. She has me try a few other exercises before telling me her opinion.

"The problem is not damage to your tongue or vocal cords. Your enemy is tension. Your voice is obstructed because you are straining to be heard and using muscle tension to force the sounds," she says.

"So then I should stop trying to sing?" I ask, half-joking.

"Again," she says and moves one octave higher on the keyboard.

I try. But I squeak and sputter and cannot make it through the first phrase. Even the cat seems to give up. It walks out of the room.

"Hear that? You are straining to get what you think is the 'right' sound. I want you to find *your* voice, not someone else's. Forget about what you think is a good voice," Gillian says, stopping her hands on the keyboard to look at me.

I'm in resistance mode.

"I don't have enough air," I protest, when Gillian asks me to lip trill Christmas carols again.

"You have the same amount of air as a Met opera singer," she says. I walk around the room a few times, thinking about this. I accidentally kick the cat, so it runs to hide under the keyboard.

I take a full breath, relax my throat completely, and try again. This time, I make it through the first verse on a single exhale.

"Girl, you have a BIG voice," she smiles.

⚶

Two days later, it is December 12. My daughter's birthday. It falls on the same date Mexicans celebrate the Virgin Mary, whom they lovingly call *La Virgen de Guadalupe*. It's an important day in Mexico; pilgrimages, parades, and dazzling fireworks are common and abundant. Hazel has adopted it as her own holiday. Every year, we join the large, Hispanic congregation in the Catholic church near our home from five in the morning until seven, when the sun comes up.

The legend goes that Guadalupe appeared to Juan Diego in rural Mexico in 1531, at sunrise. When the bishop didn't believe the story that this powerful woman would appear to a poor native, Diego unfolded his cloak. Rose petals scattered on the floor, revealing a clear image of la Virgen in a mantle made of stars, surrounded by light. Ever since then, Mexicans trust that they are under the Virgin Mary's special protection.

I wake Hazel up at four thirty. She crawls out of bed and puts her down jacket and snow boots on over her footie pajamas. We walk hand in hand, in the middle of the street, through the darkness, to the church a few blocks away. When she was younger, I wrapped her in a sleeping bag and carried her. One year, I pulled her in a sled through the heavy snow.

Hazel and I walk in silence, watching the snow sparkle under the streetlights. Everything else is dark. I lead the way past the middle school and to the top of the hill. Then as soon as we crest the hill, we hear the drumbeat, a steady boom boom boom cutting through the icy darkness. Hazel takes the lead and runs toward the dancers and music.

At the church, it feels like Hazel and I have gone through the back of a wardrobe and into a different world; one full of bright colors, lights, and the music of drums and accordions. Parking attendants do their best to find places for the steady river of Chevy pickup trucks. Men parade in through the doors and kneel to pray, wearing white jackets with sequined images of Guadalupe on the back. As soon as we sit down, children and teenagers in beaded costumes dance down the center aisle, shaking the leg rattles attached to their ankles. Hazel and I try to count the number of people awake before dawn, filling the church. Five hundred people? Four hundred, at least.

Long ago, when I am pregnant with Hazel, I go into a used furniture store looking for a bed and come home with a painting. It is a very large portrait of Guadalupe wearing a blue cape, covered in stars and surrounded by golden light. I buy it. I don't know why. I am drawn to her calm beauty.

At home, I hang the painting over the hallway in our apartment. As I do laundry or try to reason with Cole, our toddler, I talk to Guadalupe, "Can you give me a hand through bedtime? Or I may start drinking heavily and that would be bad for the baby." As my due date comes and goes without any sign of having this baby, I talk to Guadalupe nightly. It is as if she is on the other end of a phone line. I beg, "What is the baby waiting for? Can you make her come out, NOW?" When ten more days go by with no sign of labor, I say, "I'm scared. What if this baby isn't healthy? I don't know if I can handle that." She just listens quietly. At a time when I am feeling alone and unsure, Guadalupe's mature, female energy is welcome.

Hazel is born early in the morning on December 12. She comes out screaming. Minutes after she is born, I discover that it is Guadalupe Day. I watch the sunrise pink through the window and sing to this tiny baby to soothe her.

Then my dear friend Teza calls from Collingwood, Ontario. We were pregnant at the same time, but my due date was two weeks earlier and hers was a week after.

Teza says, "It's a girl!"

"I know!" I say back, confused, thinking that she is calling to congratulate me.

But she is announcing the birth of her own daughter, Rozlyn. We are two dear friends having baby girls on the same day. I picture the rays of light reaching out from Guadalupe and surrounding them both with protection.

I want to know more about the Virgin Mary, so I read up on her while I nurse. It surprises me to learn that Muslim men and women are as devoted to her as Catholics. She is the only woman mentioned by name in the Koran. In fact, her name appears more in the Koran than in the New Testament. Apparently, it's not unusual to see young Muslim women in hijab visiting the Virgin Mary at Christian shrines in Israel, for example. Muslim and Christian men and women alike speak of the Virgin's resilience and her example of love. The Virgin Mary might be the most powerful woman in the world, a true force for unity and peace.

When I received the tumor diagnosis, I prayed awkwardly to Guadalupe for help. But this is not the story of how I prayed to Guadalupe before labor, and again before my surgeries, then promised that I would go to church every week if I came out alive. No, this is the story of how I am living each day as though I may die tomorrow and, therefore, I am no longer afraid to say I believe in miracles and mystery. Before, when I talked to the painting, I was too chicken to tell anyone that I prayed to Guadalupe. I assumed my friends would smile politely, but never speak to me again.

I am not afraid anymore. Why hide it? What I've learned throughout these challenging months is that it is silly to hold back love. I still don't know where I belong spiritually; I have shopped for the right church, temple, sangha, or mosque for years. But I *do* know that I can easily, without effort or artifice, kneel before the divine presence of the Virgin Mary. She stands for love. She is for all people, no matter their background. Her compassionate gaze doesn't suggest that one way is the only way, but instead finds room for all of our beautiful brokenness.

This morning, Hazel and I stay in the church to watch the dancing and the offering of candlelight and flowers. We also stay for the singing. In our pew, Hazel and I stand between two young mothers holding infants and red roses. The babies are asleep, but the mothers are singing at full volume. They nod approvingly at Hazel as she too sings along. Hazel has this angelic voice that turns heads. The women smile and say to her, "Canta. Canta. El mundo necesita tu voz." *Sing. Sing. The world needs your voice.*

Then they pass me the booklet full of songs, as if to say, "Your daughter is joining in, singing beautifully. What's wrong with you?" Little do they know how much I squeak when I sing.

With their encouragement and Gillian's voice in my head, I open my mouth to sing. But what comes out is deep, sorrowful sobs. Once the tears start, I can't stop crying. I cry for all those who are suffering, everywhere. Then the chorus fills the church, "Madrecita, madrecita." Mother. Mother. Now I cry because I get to be Hazel's mother, as she stands next to me in her footie pajamas, singing. Then I cry because the surgeries and radiation are over. The words, "It's over. I'm OK," echo in my mind.

The minute I acknowledge the fact of those words, I feel this massive release, like when your ears clear after being plugged for hours. Only, now the feeling is in my throat. It feels clear and relaxed. Gillian is right. My vocal cords are not to blame for my lost voice. I have been holding my breath and locking my throat closed for months.

My voice did not know that it was safe to be open and vulnerable. When I lost my voice, I kept wanting to work and do exercises that would help me to get better faster. I practiced making vowel sounds in the mirror every day to strengthen my vocal cords and find my voice. Even though Gillian and the speech therapist both told me to relax, I didn't know what they meant or how to do that. *I am relaxed*, I thought. *I lie down eighty percent of the day. How can I be more relaxed?*

It takes the music and singing to loosen me up and split me open, heart first. I let emotions out that I did not know I had. I stop crying and sing. I am singing! It feels lighter than before. I let go of tension, and make room for powerful ease. Hazel says,

"Mama, you're not squeaking anymore!"

"I know. Isn't it great?"

"Well, I wouldn't say great. But it's pretty good," she says, smiling. I laugh. For the first time in months, the sound of my laughter is clear and full of joy.

24

"I can hear you when you speak! Your voice sounds strong!" Beth says enthusiastically. I am sitting in Dr. Beth Osnes's home on a very cold December morning. I had to step through two feet of snow to reach her door. Beth makes us a pot of hot tea and then bundles our feet in blankets. Beth and I are meeting because every year she travels to Guatemala to teach vocal empowerment to the same Indigenous girls I work with, who are fighting for their right for a quality education.

I've come to ask her how to empower my voice. But she wants to know how I survived my session with Gillian.

"How did the voice lesson go?" Beth asks.

I tell her about my experience in the church, and how I had no idea how much tension I was holding in my voice. Beth smiles knowingly.

She says, "When we begin with the girls in Guatemala, they are thirteen. They don't have a sense that their voice, or any part of their body, belongs to them. They don't look up, and their voices barely rise above a whisper. We have them yawn. Just a simple, wide-open yawn. Once they notice the openness and the softness at the back of the throat, then we begin. Our voices are undeniably powerful when they are open, and relaxed."

"Is there a connection between our physical voice and using our voice to take action?" I ask.

She takes a sip of her tea and says, "What I've seen around the world is that once the girls discover that their body is theirs, and that their voice is uniquely theirs, they speak up for their rights. They learn to use their voice as a tool to shape their lives."

"Does it ever go wrong?" I ask.

"Of course," says Beth. "A few years ago, a girl was assaulted on her way home from work. Her friends, my students, wanted to talk to the mayor about the need to make the streets of their town safer. But they were afraid to go to him. I helped them to do research on the number of violent incidents involving women in their town. Then they worked tirelessly to get an appointment with the mayor."

Beth pauses to pour us both another cup of tea. Then she continues,

"When we met with the mayor, he never invited us to sit down. The young, Indigenous women stood in the corner while the mayor leaned back in his oversized chair. When they gave their well-rehearsed speeches about how proud they were to live in this town and how important it was for everyone to feel safe, the mayor kept his head down and checked his messages on his phone. Then he interrupted them to say, "You think this is my problem? This is *your* problem. You are women. It's not my fault that women raise their boys to be rapists." The girls dropped their eyes to the floor, mumbled thanks, and left the building in silence.

"Did you feel like you had made a mistake?" I ask.

"I felt like I had failed completely. These young women had taken a big risk and in return, they learned how futile it was to speak up. I shouldn't have encouraged them. I should have known that you can't empower someone else, you can only empower yourself."

"What did you do?"

"I apologized to them, but they were undaunted. One young woman turned to me with a look of determination in her eyes and said, 'I thought I needed to talk to the mayor to make change. But now I know that I have to *be* the mayor.' "

I am inspired to use my voice for something bigger than myself. At home, I jump on the computer to find out how to go to the Women's March in Washington, DC. But my maximum energy level is a fraction of what it used to be, which makes travel difficult. Then I notice that there is a local march in Denver. I can do that! *Focus on what I can do, not what I can't,* I keep repeating to myself. I order a Statue of Liberty costume to wear. She represents the America I love: a safe refuge for all races, genders, and backgrounds. The point of the march, to me, is to link arms together and create the world we want, instead of being at the mercy of the winds of political change. The last time I marched was in 2004, for women's reproductive rights. *Why had I stopped making my voice heard?*

Life got in the way. With babies and fulltime work, I could barely find enough time to shower, much less become an activist. But my perfectionism also got in the way. I was always searching for the single, right way to get involved with issues that I cared about. I wanted a guarantee that my efforts would make an impact. And I didn't want to risk losing the approval of my family or friends by joining the "wrong" movement. So I didn't do anything, because I didn't know how to move forward. But the world can't wait while I try to get it perfect. I want to join in the fun of making the world better now. It helps to remember that I don't have to single-handedly make change in the world.

As Beth said to me before I left her home the other day, "Speaking up and taking action is not about planting a flag and declaring greatness. It is about letting go of the single-author narrative that we must change the world on our own. We all need significant help from others."

≈

On Saturday, January 21, 2017, a dozen friends and I gather to raise our voices in the Women's March in Denver. Natasha, Alli, and

Teza, my childhood friends, send messages to cheer us on. My friend Tania shows up in a Statue of Liberty costume too, and carries a sign that says, "My friend's life was saved by a Syrian immigrant." She is referring to me and Dr. Al-Mefty. I am moved that she is awake before dawn, in a ridiculous costume, willing to take a stand.

We come around the corner of one street and there are anti-march protestors on the sidewalk, shouting, "You lost the election! Go home!" But I don't feel a need to react or shout back. I just keep walking and smiling. The difference between when I felt full of rage and now is that I am channeling my energy into something I am *for*, instead of raging at everything I am *against*. I remember what my yoga teacher, Sukhraj, said, "Step into the wind and transform your negativity into something good and positive." *I am linking arms with others and stepping into the wind.* I feel privileged to walk with my daughter and so many beautiful women, men, and children in a sea of peaceful dissent. At one intersection, we are bottlenecked and moving slowly in the crowd. A stranger leans over to me and says, "It doesn't feel like we are making any progress."

"Oh, but we are!" I say enthusiastically. "A couple of months ago," I tell her, "I couldn't even walk to the bathroom!" She looks confused. Then she laughs, and seems genuinely satisfied with my answer. In my head, I come up with the secret pathways to being brave:

- Aim for progress, not perfection

- Focus on what you can do, not what you can't

- Collaborate, don't compare and compete

- Feel the fear, and do it anyway

The next day, the newspaper shows photos of women's marches around the world. The images of women in New Delhi and Guatemala City move me to tears. Thousands of women, inspired by the marches in the US, flood the streets, holding signs that say, "I will go out!" They are demanding safe public spaces. They want to walk home without being harassed or raped. They are making their voices heard.

A woman using her voice to stand up for what she believes inspires countless others to use their voices, around the world. This is why it matters to speak up. Every time a woman makes her voice heard, another woman is listening, is speaking up, and is taking a stand.

In bed that night, I write down in my journal, *I am a woman, a mother, and an immigrant who wants to lift my community out of anxiety and fear. I don't want to wait any longer to find the right way to do this. I spent too much time in my life trying to get it right, to please others, and to keep pain and struggle at bay. The world needs me to be brave enough to try, to iterate, and to expand the limits of what is possible. The only thing getting in the way is that I get stuck trying to find the single, right way. There is no one way. There is no guarantee of safety. When I focus on the outcome, I get paralyzed by all the things that could go wrong. I want to focus on making progress. Even if I can't speak very loudly, I will use my voice on paper and in the streets. I want to inspire others to let courage, not caution, be their guide.*

25

It's been nine months since our lives were turned upside down by this brainstem tumor, and lately I am having a tough time trusting in the unknown. Since the type of tumor that I have is incurable, I live in a state of perpetual uncertainty. *Is the tumor dormant, active, or growing enormous again in my skull?* My next follow-up with the doctors is two months away.

Until then, I meditate, write, and try to trust that the universe has my back. But I have many sleepless nights, wondering what my future holds. I go to see Michael, my therapist.

Begin scene. Light falls through the room as Susie sits on the couch, looking down at her hands. Michael sits opposite, a notepad poised on his lap.

"I'm anxious. If I knew what the doctors were going to say, I could feel empowered and healed," I complain.

"Forget about the doctors. Why not feel empowered and healed now?"

"Because the tumor could be growing!"

"Or, it could be shrinking. What is the harm in picturing a positive future?"

"My mind prefers worst-case scenarios."

"You have come so far. What is the proof that you won't weather the next storm as well as you have weathered the last one?"

"That I am scared and feel helpless."

"You know, feeling helpless and terrified does not better prepare you for anything. How about leaving room for mystery?"

"How do I do that?"

"Try raising the vibration. Picture yourself in your fullest, most enlivened state."

"That's my point; I'm having a tough time accessing that right now."

"Well, I can see you giving an interview on TV in the future, saying, 'I'm so grateful I healed. I get how powerful we are. I can't believe that was ten years ago.' "

"Ha! But do you really think that's in the realm of possibility?"

"Why not? Once you embrace the unknown, and let go of believing all your negative thoughts, things happen that you've never experienced before. Try again. Who are you in the future?"

"I'm healthy. I trust life. I feel safe being me, and I don't hold back love. I am a good-news story that represents what is possible. I help people move beyond fear."

"Now you're talking! And what do you want people to know?"

"We're not just good enough as we are, we're incredible. And, we have powerful voices that have no limits."

"Yes! The truth of what the future holds for us is unknown. And one way to imagine the unknown is dark. But when people embrace the highest possibility for themselves, they do better."

"I think I just need practice trusting the unknown."

"How could you do that?"

⁂

I leave Michael's office with his question still alive in my mind. On the bulletin board in the waiting room is a picture of a tent on a beach. I have a crazy idea, suddenly. I go home and design a vacation with my family that leaves plenty of room for uncertainty.

We fly to Mexico. When Kurt, the kids, and I step off the plane, we have no idea where we will sleep that night. We have a map. We have a few tips from friends scribbled on a notepad. We rent a minivan from a super-enthusiastic young woman at the airport who keeps calling me "lovely lady." We have sleeping bags and I have an inflatable pillow to support my neck fusion that I cling to like a security blanket. We know we want to camp in the two tents we have with us, but where? *Is it safe? What will we eat? What will we do?*

We have one phone with a Mexico data plan for route-finding and emergencies. The kids have no screens. They entertain themselves on the long drives by blowing into empty glass Coke bottles.

Twenty years ago, before cell phones and Google, Kurt and his friend Scott kayaked the entire length of Baja, Mexico along the Sea of Cortez. It was a two-month journey steeped in trust and the slow pace of a hand-powered boat. They moved through a curious new landscape with Cardón cacti as tall as trees, frigate birds with seven-foot wingspans soaring overhead, and flying fish slapping them in the face as they paddled. At night, they pulled their kayaks ashore and ate whatever the locals had to offer. That was in 1997, and it was the last time Kurt was here. The kids and I have never been to Baja. The US State Department's website urges us to reconsider our travel plans because of the risk of violent crimes in the area. "We cannot guarantee your safety," the site warns.

We open the map at the gas station and look for a place to sleep. We notice a sheltered bay on the east coast, out of the wind and away from other spring break tourists. But we don't have enough daylight to make it to the coast, so we look for a place to sleep inland. We hear there is a waterfall about an hour and a half away. But we don't know where.

"Things have changed a little since 1997," announces Kurt when we have been driving on a dirt road with no road signs for over an hour. I imagine us stranded in the desert.

"Does a cactus hold water in its trunk?" I ask Kurt.

"Not really," says my biologist husband. "You have to pummel their pulp for a long time and chew on it, spines and all, to get any water."

I look out the window at endless dry desert and the setting sun. I think about how crazy it is to deliberately bring my family into the unknowns of this risky landscape.

Just as I am about to ask Kurt to turn around, we make it to the end of the road. A tall, local man with a cowboy hat and handlebar mustache stands there like a mirage, and greets us warmly in Spanish.

"I am Prisciliano Elehazar de la Peña Ruíz. Would your family like to rest? I have cabins you can rent near the waterfall."

I want to kiss him.

Each day, we don't know what we will find at the end of the next dirt road. Cole says, "I know we're getting close to something good when the minivan door squeaks like crazy." What he means is, when we leave the paved road for the dirt, the bumps in the road shake the whole van. I thank my little inflatable pillow for softening the blows; I always find a way to sit in the car comfortably, without rattling my neck or head. After several teeth-chattering kilometers, each evening we arrive somewhere spectacular with white sand, green water, mangrove trees, ibis birds, islands to snorkel around, and generous, gentle locals.

One night we sleep on a beach in a town with a sign that says "población: 41." But we only count seven people. In the morning, we wake to find over thirty donkeys lingering outside our tents. Maybe the donkeys were counted in the population census. Another time, we hear of hot springs up the next canyon, but the beach "road" to arrive there vanishes at high tide. There are no nearby stores or restaurants. We have one rule: our food must be caught or found. Kurt teaches the kids how to spearfish and they hunt for our dinner. Meanwhile, I chat up the locals to find out who the best fishermen are and if I can buy fish from them. Let's just say I like to have a solid back-up plan. Every evening, we eat barred snapper and triggerfish tacos, either caught by Kurt or bought from the back of a truck. We cook them on our backcountry stove, overlooking the sea.

At night, we wash our fish bones back into the ocean and look at the stars. Before this trip, the kids only knew two constellations: the Big Dipper and Orion. On this vacation, the kids learn over thirty constellations, and make up many more of their own. They are so engaged in their surroundings that Cole has me set an alarm for midnight so he can try to see the Southern Cross, while Hazel has fun inventing a giant, three-tentacled octopus constellation.

"Show me how you made all the stars fit into something new," I say, lying down next to Hazel, looking up.

"I didn't do anything. They just go together," she says.

I look and look. It takes me a while, but I finally see invisible lines that link the stars into an octopus.

"See how everything is connected, Mama? Don't you see how everything just belongs together?" she asks. With time, I do.

When I look at the sky with wonder, I don't feel small or unworthy anymore. I feel giant. Everything is connected. We all belong here.

I settle down in the sand to sleep, and take in this beautiful world of stars and sea and family. When we talk about the unknown, I usually picture the edge of a cliff or a dark cave. But the unknown is also what the stars are to me, what whale song is to me, and bird migration. It's northern lights and salmon journeying home. It's a hummingbird's heartbeat, the design of a spider web, and the way life grows from an egg. It's falling in love, having a baby, and raising a family.

I don't pretend to understand the world. In fact, I am partial to its mysteries. I prefer to look about in wonder, to bow down in humility, and to kneel down in gratitude. On this secluded beach in Mexico, the unknown is beautiful to me again. It is possibility. I don't know where I'll be tomorrow, or how I'll feel in the morning, but it matters less and less. I remember that there is a plan. There always has been; it's just not mine.

26

A close friend of mine, Sara, is dying. That, plus a scheduled check-up with my doctor next month, has me thinking about time and how best to spend it. In the morning, I wake up and throw myself into the future. At night, I go to bed, nostalgic for the past morning, wanting to do the day over again, better. It's like I am bungee-jumping from the future to the past. I can stay focused on the here and now, but only for a few minutes. If a genie appeared to grant me three wishes, I am embarrassed to admit that they might all have to do with time. 1) Can I roll it back just a little? 2) Tell me, how much do I have left? 3) What is the most meaningful way to spend my time on this planet? But I don't need a genie. My friend Sara is showing me the way.

I find out that Sara is in hospice after seven years of battling a malignant cancer that spread from her chest to her brain. I want to go to her, but I don't know if she wants to see me. After all, I haven't been available to her since I got sick. Plus, I'm scared. I am uncomfortable around death and dying. It is too close to home. I want to be surrounded by survival stories. I don't want to say goodbye to someone I love. My friend Catherine picks me up and drives me to Sara's house anyway. There isn't time to say, "No, thanks. Not today."

Once inside Sara's home, everything changes. I am desperate to see her. I practically run up the stairs to her room, tripping over their cat on the way. Catherine and I push open the door and see Sara smiling, her eyes bright, fussing over where we're going to sit.

We come to give her our attention, but all she wants to do is give us love. She even has presents for us. Mine is a t-shirt to help me face my terminal illness. In purple cursive, it says, "CHALLENGE ACCEPTED. I

GOT THIS." This knocks me to my knees. I fight back the tears and put the t-shirt on. It fits perfectly.

Then she wants to talk about cakes. Sara has always loved good food. She describes in mouth-watering detail her favorites: Triple layer chocolate cake. Decadent flourless chocolate explosion. Flourless chocolate cake with white-chocolate ganache. She moves right into describing her favorite cheeses, the soft bries and camemberts they sell at the cheese shop around the corner. Catherine and I sit and listen, our stomachs growling.

"Can you take an order?" Sara asks, and looks at us as if we are dumb not to bring paper and a pen when visiting her.

"Sure. What would you like?" Catherine asks while I scramble to find something to write with.

"No. This isn't for me," Sara says. "I want you to bring special cakes to my family and friends, to thank them for me."

As I scribble down Sara's cake order for her loved ones on the back of my hand, all I can think is that this is so Sara. She lives and dies from a place of joy and gratitude.

The following Monday, a huge snowstorm hits our town. The cherry and crabapple trees that had already blossomed are now bowed low, as if grieving. On Tuesday morning, the world is quieter under the snow, but also full of light. The phone rings. Sara has died.

I am bereft of poise and strength. Sara was so alive at our last visit; how could she be gone? Life is fragile, frail even. One minute I am running along a high mountain trail, jumping over creeks in the sunshine. The next minute I am in a neurosurgeon's office. One minute Sara is dancing with me to "Girls Just Wanna Have Fun," the next she is gone. Outside it has started to rain, melting the snow.

I keep walking around my house in circles, unsure of what to do. Luckily, I remember that Catherine and I have direct orders, not just from Sara, but from the universe. Buy cakes. Hand deliver them. It doesn't make any sense. Sara is not here to direct us. Nobody really expects or needs cake. But it is a beautiful impulse. How can we not listen and act?

The orders tell me to practice tolerating uncertainty. Get comfortable listening to the improbable. My logical brain says there is no point. Or is there? After all, Sara beat the odds the doctors gave her again and again. Maybe she is telling me that I can live a long and healthy life if I believe in a universe that isn't just about disease and disasters, but also about unreasonable, improbable acts of love and generosity.

Catherine plans the delivery route while I go to the bakery. I order every chocolate cake in the display case. José, working behind the counter, asks, "Are you celebrating?"

"Yes." I say, because he's right. We are.

The next thing I know, we are peering through screen doors, as if it is totally normal for two middle-aged women to show up with a cake box on your doorstep. We stumble over a few introductions, then say awkwardly, "Sara really wanted you to have this triple-layer chocolate cake with chocolate buttercream frosting." We don't know what to expect in terms of reactions. After all, we are intruding at a tough time.

Sara's mom looks at us, then the cake, and a big smile spreads across her face. Then she says, "So she told you to get cakes, eh? She told me to get gorgeous cheeses for each of her nurses."

Many people at the end of their lives go fighting and full of regrets. Not Sara. Every day until her last, she woke up wondering, How can I give love and spread joy today? She challenges me to show up on others' doorsteps to say thank you. To say, "Remember to celebrate, no matter what." It may not be rational, but it feels like the best way to live.

Today, Sara reminds me to unclip time's bungee rope, stop worrying about the future, and concentrate on where I am, which happens to be with Sara's mom and sister, eating a triple-layer chocolate cake with buttercream frosting. This is beautiful right here, right now. There is a lot to celebrate.

⚜

In a few weeks, I'll travel to Boston with Kurt for follow-up doctor's appointments. The remaining bits of tumor in my skull are likely dormant and should stay that way for decades. Yet there is this unpleasant game of being scanned every few months to see if things are quiet or spreading. Between those scans, my doctor says, "Live your normal life." But it's difficult to relax. *Am I going to die young?*

When we travel to Boston, Dr. Liebsch will order pictures of my skull and neck for the first time since radiation ended. I see myself put on the hospital gown, sit on the cold examining table, and watch the contrast liquid get injected into my arm. I hear the technicians snap down the fiberglass mask over my mouth and nose to keep my head still, and slide me into the MRI machine. I know that the knocks and bells of the machine will ring out bad news or good news.

In my imagination, my doctor turns to me and says, "Looks good. See you in six months!" Then again, he might turn to me and say, "I'm sorry, but the tumor is growing." It's hard not to beg. *Please let me have a clean scan. Please don't make me tell my children that I am going to die, that the surgery and radiation didn't work.*

Every time I cling to how *I* want things to be in life, the universe gives me a lesson in letting go of control.

One evening, Kurt comes home from work and says, "I need to go to Tucson to help my parents get rid of their stuff."

"I'll go with you."

"Are you sure?"

"I feel strong. It'll be fun."

My in-laws, Rick and MJ, hold on to everything. They are not hoarders, exactly. They are wonderful people who feel safe surrounded by objects that they might need someday, like enough ace bandages to mummify a horse, and dozens of cardboard boxes in all sizes and shapes.

The problem is that the rest of us don't know something valuable when we see it. "Why would anyone throw these away?" asks MJ, as she reorganizes a leaning tower of salt packets from Olive Garden. She stacks them in the cupboard next to a rotary-dial telephone and an antique cheese grater that doesn't grate cheese anymore.

They hold on to food, too. On this visit, MJ hands me a yogurt.

"Wait. This one is expired by a few months," I say.

"It's fine. The expiration date is just a suggestion," she says, and waves me off like I am a fly.

Once, Rick was so sick he couldn't get out of bed.

"Do you think it's the flu?" Kurt asked.

"No, I'm pretty sure I ate something bad," answered Rick in a hoarse whisper.

"How do you know?"

"Well, there were hot dogs sitting out for a while. I ate one and it tasted a little off."

"But you ate it anyway?" asked Kurt.

"Yeah. But the second one was even worse," said Rick, unphased.

When we arrive in Tucson, ready to swoop in and save the day, the joke's on us. MJ and Rick's home is spacious and spotless. They worked for weeks to de-clutter, letting go of *almost* everything. In the process, they found out what they want to do with their time. Rick wants to rebuild his old Jeep. MJ wants to write her life stories for her grandchildren.

Instead of cleaning, we spend the weekend sitting and walking together, just happy to be in one another's company. We eat pie, watch a nesting pair of hawks, and tell stories that make us laugh so hard that some of us pee our pants. It's a gift to be able to focus on our relationship, instead of on all that stuff.

Back at home, I am inspired. If they can do it, so can I! I start with the tangle of ancient ski gear, ice skates, and hockey sticks, then turn my attention to the overstuffed bookcases, bathroom cupboards, and bedroom closets. It's easy to let go of the old, and the no-longer-useful, but it's tough to let go of gifts and treasures I once loved: a jacket I won in a race, the jewelry box I was given at graduation, a book of Annie Dillard essays. I keep moving them out of the "donate" pile and back into the closet. When I finally let them go, I feel a weight lift from my shoulders.

I keep going. I want to make the things I love more visible and let go of everything else. I pay my son to go through thousands of photos on our computer and make eight photo books with one hundred photos each; one book for each of the last eight years. I frame and hang the very best pictures and delete the rest. The idea is simple: spend time enjoying life instead of organizing it.

With all of this tidying up, I wonder, *Am I spring cleaning or am I preparing for death?*

For now, I'm accepting that at some point I will die and I will not need all this stuff. Nor do I want to leave it for my children to have to manage. Letting go implies loss, but I am not letting go of this life. I'm letting go of control and materialism. The change feels really good. Before, I was trying to hold on to as much as I possibly could. I wanted to hermetically seal moments of health and happiness. Now, I'm able to put good things out the door, because I recognize that there is more goodness where it came from. Meanwhile, the stuff isn't lifting me up, it's weighing me down.

But it takes me one more lesson in letting go of things to truly feel free.

I have a red, woven bracelet around my right wrist. It's really just three threads braided together into a single red cord, no thicker than a hair tie. It was given to me by my Cambodian friend, Cho. He had it blessed by a monk to wish me safety and health on my journeys ahead.

Every morning, I study the red, thinning threads like lines on my palm. I am somehow convinced that possessing the bracelet is what gives me vitality. *Is the red cord still there? Good. I'm alive.*

Then yesterday, my son Cole and I are out for a walk. When I look down at my wrist, the red bracelet is gone. Cole drops to his hands and knees to search for it; he knows how important it is to me. But I have a strange sense of relief. It is gone, but I am still standing. I am no longer counting on something external to tell me how I feel on the inside.

"Don't worry," I say. "Let it be."

"Are you sure?" he asks.

"Yeah. Why?"

"Because you haven't taken your eyes off the ground."

Cole's right. Even though I feel relieved and ready to let go, there's a part of me that still believes that I need something external for strength. I call my friend Christine again, for advice. "Red cords are supposed to break," she explains when I tell her about my bracelet. "When it's gone, it means that you are a different person who has integrated the insights you needed to learn."

Life is fragile, but it is also rich, and I am resilient. I shift from anticipating a bad report from the doctors to remembering that facing death has brought me clarity and joy in the past year. *I don't feel loss, I feel amazing. I have unbreakable support and love. I can come through this better than before.*

27

It is my birthday. I am forty-six years old. I made it another year, a whole lap around the sun. I don't take that for granted. Last year, I celebrated my birthday by running on a mountain trail, winning the masters division of an ultramarathon, just two weeks before my diagnosis. This year, we celebrate by going to see my doctors. My birthday just happens to coincide with my follow-up appointments in Boston where they'll take several MRI images of my brain and cervical spine to see if there is any new tumor activity.

Leading up to this moment, I have worried about the outcome of these doctors' visits. In the bad version, the doctors tell me, "I'm sorry. The tumor has grown and your body cannot handle any more surgery or radiation. There is nothing we can do." *Will I go quickly? Or will it be slow and painful?* These thoughts don't surprise me; they are always there with their sharp brightness, like a trumpet solo in a mariachi song. I don't like them; I don't like discomfort. I want to know that I am healthy and fine so I can exhale. I don't just *want* a good outcome, I *need* it.

In the good version, the doctors say, "Good news! The surgeries and radiation worked!" But I spin on the bad outcome at night, lying awake. Fear hisses at me, "You shouldn't go to Boston. You know it's going to be bad news."

I decide to try something different. I talk to Fear. This is a trick I learn from Elizabeth Gilbert's wonderful book, *Big Magic*. Once Gilbert recognizes that her fear is the most boring thing about her, she stops trying to fight it off. Instead, she relaxes and addresses her fear with calm indifference. She even invites it to join her wherever she goes, but forbids it to drive. I try a similar approach.

"Fear," I say. "Thank you for caring about me. I know that you are just trying to keep me safe. But I am going to Boston. You are welcome to come with me, because I know you would anyway, even if I didn't invite you. But until then, I am the only one who decides what to do, what not to do, and how to live." It feels silly to talk out loud to my fear, especially when I notice that Kurt and the kids can hear me. But it also feels empowering. Fear's hold over me wobbles, shakes, then falls, while my own voice gains clarity and power.

In the rehearsal of all possible outcomes, I don't expect what happens in Boston.

While Kurt spends hours in hospital waiting rooms, I do my best impersonation of a perfectly-still person inside the MRI and the CT scanners. The technicians take dozens of images of my brain and neck that the radiologists and doctors will examine. These images are their most sophisticated tools for knowing what's going on inside my skull. They hold the answers to the status of the tumor remnants that could not be safely removed a year ago, the ones that were radiated for eight weeks.

All I can do now is wait. I sit on the crinkly paper on Dr. Al-Mefty's examining table and listen for the sound of his squeaky shoes walking down the hall to my room. Kurt sits quietly on a chair by the window. I hear footsteps in the hall, but they stop and turn into the room next to ours. How many patients will this doctor see today? How many times will he say, "I'm sorry. There is nothing more we can do for you."

The minutes tick by slowly, painfully. Finally, I hear his squeaky shoes get closer. Dr. Al-Mefty enters the room with Dr. Arnaout. It takes both of them several more minutes to figure out how to open the files with the images of my skull on the computer. Then they squint at the screen and say nothing for a long, long time. I look over their shoulder and see my brain in sharp black and white contrast. Looking at an

MRI scan is not so different from looking at an X-ray; there are the tidy white bones and the mysterious black space around them. Only, now you can also see white blurry shapes that are tissues. All those layers of muscle, blood, and scar tissue cloud the picture substantially. I have no idea what I am looking at, but I stare intently anyway, as if it will make sense to me somehow.

The way they squint at the images, I assume they are seeing something terrible and don't know how to tell me.

"What do you see?" I ask, nervously.

"Hard to say what those blobs are," says Dr. Arnaout.

"Blobs? What do you mean?"

"See those white puffy blobs? We can't tell if they are scar tissue or tumor."

"You don't know?" I ask incredulously. After all, Dr. Al-Mefty is one of the world's leading experts on skull-base tumors.

"Well, one radiologist report says the tumor is bigger. Another report says it is smaller. To me, the tumor looks to be the same size. Maybe smaller." says Dr. Al-Mefty.

"Isn't there a way to measure it precisely?" Kurt speaks up.

"It's just too hard to tell what is tumor and what isn't with all of the scar tissue in there. We don't know. We need more images for comparison," says Dr. Arnaout.

"What do we do now?"

"Nothing. We'll see you again in six months."

I am stunned. I had vividly imagined receiving the best news ever. And I had rehearsed my response to the worst news ever. I thought, either way, at least we would know. It never occurred to me that I would walk away from today with the same news and the same level of uncertainty. The doctors shrug and stare some more at the images.

"Well. How do you feel?" asks Dr. Al-Mefty.

"Great!" I say truthfully.

"How is your voice now?" He asks, with serious curiosity.

"Stronger than it has ever been," I say and smile.

"How you feel is our best indication. Go have a beautiful summer. You get to keep that smile," says Dr. Al-Mefty.

I want to, but I can't quite access that place of confidence to go have a beautiful summer. I need a definitive answer.

We take a taxi across town to Mass General hospital to meet with my radiation oncologist, Dr. Liebsch. Maybe he will have the answer that I need to feel safe. When we arrive, he is all business. For thirty minutes, he conducts a thorough physical and mental exam. I stick out my tongue, walk in a straight line, answer one hundred questions, try to turn my neck as far as I can to the left and to the right, touch my toes, and touch each of my fingers with my thumbs. I cannot tell if I am doing well on any of these tests. He doesn't say anything. And his serious expression doesn't change.

Dr. Liebsch rarely smiles. Last fall, I wore a Star Trek captain costume to my appointment with him, because I thought the radiation room looked like a flight deck. I thought it might make him laugh. But he didn't say anything about my outfit. He just kept examining me without ever cracking a grin.

Finally, Dr. Liebsch pauses and says in his thick German accent, "No radiation damage. No brain deficiencies. Neck fusion is holding strong."

"That's good, right?" I ask.

"Very goot. Yah," he says, with cool composure.

"But what about the report that says the tumor is bigger," I ask.

"That radiologist is very cautious. He always says that," Dr. Liebsch says, waving his hand dismissively.

"What about the report that says it is smaller?" I push a little.

"Yah. And the one that says it is the same. I've seen them all. So now you get to choose."

"What do you mean?"

"Forget about the reports for a moment. How do you feel?" he asks sternly.

"Great," I say for the second time today, and mean it.

"You want me to tell you how you are. But I can't tell you that with the certainty that you want. Focus on how you feel. Listen when I tell you that you passed the physical exam with flying colors. It's up to you; choose the report you want," Dr. Liebsch says, and pats me on the shoulder. Then he gestures to let me know that my medical gown is still wide open.

As I stumble to fix my stupid gown, I get the giggles. I can't stop laughing. It feels like I am exhaling for the first time in a year. I am the expert of my life!

For months, I have been waiting for doctors to tell me how I am. But now the neurosurgeons say that I am the only one who can know that. The image I had of the doctor walking into the room, smiling, and saying, "Go! Be free. You have a clean bill of health!" might only be the stuff of movies. In my experience, it is more likely that the doctor will say, "I don't know." The only thing I can count on is the steadiness of uncertainty.

Kurt and I walk out of the hospital into the sunshine, now sharp and beautiful because of the mix of dark clouds around it.

This is what I know: I am going to live. For at least the next seven minutes, anyway, before we get in a car and drive on the freeway. I know, too, that I am going to die.

This is all any of us ever know. But we can live like that, one day at a time. We stop trying to keep up with the world's expectations of us. We start paying attention to the truth of who we are. We savor each delicious moment, and we walk with each other through discomfort. When adversity strikes, we delight in the unknown. Because in mystery there is choice, and there is joy.

The Steadiness of Uncertainty

I am not the person I used to be. I am much happier. This is not what I expected when the doctors gave me that scary diagnosis. Once I questioned the belief that my value came from outside sources, my voice felt unshackled, and my depression lifted. Now I know that worth is something we are born with, not something we need to earn.

The world needs us to be fierce enough to see challenges as gifts, to choose brave over perfect, to express our unique selves, and to expand the limits of what is possible. The only thing getting in the way is that we get stuck trying to find our way out of pain and discomfort. There is no way to avoid uncertainty. There is no guarantee of safety.

To step into our infinite power:

- *Redefine the rules together.* Let's make our homes, schools, and organizations places where it is safe, even expected, to take risks. Instead of relying on unspoken expectations, let's create new ground rules together. Before an important meeting, have each person answer these questions, borrowed from Priya Parker's *The Art of Gathering*: "What do you need to feel safe to express yourself? What do you need to be willing to take a risk in this conversation today?"

- *Build a culture of courage, not competition.* Find the people who are doing good work and join them. Our ambition is a beautiful thing when it propels us to be the highest version of ourselves and to cheer on others who are working to do the same. It starts to sour when we are looking over our shoulder and wondering who will be interviewed first by Oprah. As the vocal empowerment coach Dr. Beth Osnes says, "Speaking up and taking action is not about planting a flag and declaring greatness. It's about letting go of the single-author narrative that we must change the world on our own." We are trained to think we must be better than those around us to succeed. But in my experience, the path to lasting fulfillment is paved in generosity and collaboration.

- *A year to live.* Imagine that you only have twelve months to live. How would you behave? No one should need to undergo a major crisis in order to rethink their priorities and remember the preciousness of life. Your imagination is powerful. Use it to create a sense of urgency. Act as if this is the only life you have to live, because it is.

- *Raise the vibration.* Our view of what is possible is often too small, and our frequency is too low to manifest what we really want. Play is purpose: give yourself permission to play and big things will happen. When I was struggling to think optimistically, I came upon these words hand painted on a signpost: "BIG up. Live up. Tune up. *Way* up." They remind me to check my "spirit-o-meter" and raise it a couple of notches. I do this by asking one question, How can I give love and spread joy today?

QUESTIONS FOR DISCUSSION AND REFLECTION

Introduction

Susie seemed to have it all: a beautiful family, leadership of a great company, medals as a champion ultrarunner. She was even the Dalai Lama's personal guide on a visit to the US. But it never felt like enough. No one, not even her closest friends, knew she was struggling with anxiety and depression. She tried to drown out her feelings with more accomplishments. But there were consequences to straining to do everything perfectly. Her health was at risk. At forty-five years old, she was diagnosed with a rare form of cancer in her skull. Several neurosurgeons gave her an immediate death sentence. The diagnosis sparked the question, "If you come out of this unharmed, how are you going to live?" Susie realized that her strategy of striving, performing, and pretending wasn't working anymore. She had a choice, and wrote down how she wanted to move forward, "I choose joy over fear, and brave over perfect."

After thirty-six consecutive hours of surgery on her skull, Susie walked into a new life. The only problem? She physically lost her voice. In *Fierce Joy*, Susie finds her true voice, lets go of anxiety over what she *should* do, and becomes who she was meant to be.

Fierce Joy is the inspiring story of an ordinary woman fighting for her life and reclaiming her voice. But it is also a cautionary tale of what happens when we shrink our voices with perfectionism, and a call-to-action to express our full, unique selves.

This discussion guide is designed to help us find our voices in these challenging times, together.

Part I

1. Susie doesn't think she is a perfectionist because her house is messy and she wears pajamas to the grocery store. She writes, "But I never believe I am good enough…I want to find the single, right way beyond criticism to success." (Page 8) What does perfectionism mean to you? In what ways might you be a perfectionist?

2. "Women are praised for their beauty or their extraordinary accomplishments. When we don't feel beautiful and when we aren't the top performer, we don't question our culture's values, we question our worth." (Page 13.) At a young age, Susie internalized that she must prove her value to earn a place in the world. What other messages are girls receiving about their worth? What about boys? How else can we define success beyond accolades and accomplishments?

3. When Susie attends an elite college, she feels like an imposter. "I am convinced that I don't deserve to be here. I don't have what it takes." (Page 23.) Have you ever felt like an imposter? What helped you to overcome that feeling?

4. Susie's therapist says, "Our culture sends a clear message to women: good mothers are calm, loving, and willingly sacrifice themselves for their children. When you fall short of those expectations, the problem isn't that we have created an unattainable myth of mothering, but that you are a failure." (Page 37.) The myth of the good mother causes Susie to feel like she is broken. What myth of the "good parent" did you grow up believing? How does that myth (or another one) make you feel like a failure sometimes?

5. Have you ever kept a list in your mind of what constitutes the perfect romantic partner? What qualities did you include, or do you still include?

Part II

1. Susie defines "voice" as the instrument we use to express our deepest feelings and our unique selves. "I feel lucky to be born in a time and place where I am free to speak out. But that doesn't mean I have always known how to find my voice and use it to author my life." (Page 58.) Can you remember a time when you found your voice and expressed yourself freely? When was that? How could you amplify your inner voice?

2. Kurt says to Susie before she spends three days alone, "We're all going to die. The question is, How do you want to live?" How might you answer that question?

3. Asking for help is not usually in a perfectionist's vocabulary, or anyone's, really. One reason Susie is afraid to reach out is that she doesn't want to be a burden to others. Can you think of a time when a friend asked you for help? How did you feel being asked? Did your opinion of that friend change for the worse?

4. "The worst thing is to die without knowing yourself." What do you think of those words offered by the Dalai Lama? If you knew that you were loved, how would you act? What would it look like to be unapologetically yourself?

5. Write a letter to your daughter, son, or someone important to you. What do you wish you had known growing up? What kind of bravery did you need when you were their age?

Part III

1. Susie loses her voice after her operations. She says, "So this is the taste of voicelessness: bitter isolation, acidic futility, burning determination. I took my voice for granted. Never again." p. __ When have you ever felt voiceless? How do you take your voice for granted?

2. What kind of mother did you want? What kind of mother did you get? What do you appreciate about who she is or was? How could you appreciate who *you* are more?

3. "Beware of hope," writes Susie's therapist. "You can't feel at peace if what you hope for is not happening." (Page 139.) What is the alternative to hope, according to the therapist?

4. On the fall equinox, Susie thinks, "The way our culture emphasizes balance makes me feel like I should figure out how to be more physically, mentally, and spiritually poised every. single. day." What is your relationship with trying to find a work/life balance? Has your desire for balance ever caused you more stress rather than less?

Part IV

1. One morning, Susie wakes up full of rage. She is tired of feeling that the world is not safe, and tired of being motivated by fear. But she says "good girls don't express rage." Ultimately, she sits with her feelings. "Before, I thought I was brave because I pushed past pain. But bravery is facing fear, being vulnerable, and sitting in discomfort with anger." (Page 160.) What message did you receive about expressing anger? What do you do when you feel angry?

2. "When I aim my perfectionism at myself, it's about not being good enough...But when I turn my gaze outward, my perfectionism is about everyone and everything else not being good enough. It's all about control." (Page 170.) In what areas of your life do you prefer to be in control? How do you act when you believe that you are right and others are wrong?

3. The young, Indigenous girls in Guatemala inspire Susie to use her voice for something bigger than herself. She writes, "[Before], I wanted a guarantee that my efforts would make an impact...But the world can't wait while I try to get it perfect. I want to join in the fun of making the world better now."

(Page 187.) Who inspires you to take action? If you focus on what you can do, not what you can't, what might you do to take action now?

4. To make friends with the unknown, Susie designs a vacation with no plans. She doesn't know where she will sleep each night. When was the last time you went on a trip without a plan? How comfortable are you with the unknown, especially in terms of your health or money?

ACKNOWLEDGMENTS

I am deeply grateful to the following people for bringing this book out of hiding and into the world. Thank you…

For bedrock support: Marilyn Caldwell, Douglas Caldwell, Janet Leslie, MJ and Rick Rinehart, Judy and Wilmot Matthews, Ellen and Bob Wright, Gail and Bob Farquharson, Judy Korthals, Brooke and Dan Neidich, Theresa and Scott Beck

For extended family: Faith Catlin and John Griesemer, Deb and Pat Barnes, Comfort and Kit Halsey Leckerling, Missy and Alden Smith, Sue and Jack Kruse, Linda and Tom Cole

For sisterhood: Rachel Brown, Allison Dancy, Diane Rinehart, Natasha Taylor, Allison Talacko, Teza Lawrence, Jill Sivers

For brotherhood: Jake Caldwell, Derek Caldwell, Rick Rinehart, Blair Dancy

For guardian angels: Lisa Korthals, Sara Lacopo, Chris Korthals

For mentorship: Rick Ridgeway, Christine Carter

For innovative publishing and creative brilliance: Chris McKenney, Natasha Vera, Brenda Knight, Lee Oglesby, Yaddyra Peralta, Hannah Jorstad Paulsen, Michelle Lewy, and the entire team at Mango

For refuge and quiet: Deborah Briggs, Polly Hoppin and Bob Thomas, Karen and Dan Taylor, Robin and Ward Brown, The Seybolt family, Vickie and Bob Cunningham, John Roemer, Phyllis Rogers and Mark Weakley

For healing: Michael Vladeck, Sukhraj Kaur Gipple, Orianne Evans, Mia Seymour, Katie Andrews, Danae Shanti, Taylor Moffitt White, Juliette Reynolds, Dr. Mary Shackelton, Dr. Jennifer Christensen

For medical genius: Dr. Ossama Al-Mefty, Dr. Norbert Liebsch, Dr. Omar Arnaout, Dr. John Chi, Sarajune Dagen, Kristen Ambrose, Dr. Rick Rinehart, Dr. Moustapha Abou-Samra

For inspiration: The children of the Burr Proton Beam Therapy Center at MGH, Mel Stewart, Jesse Rothman, Joaquin LaGrave-Stewart

For editing honesty and solidarity: John Griesemer, Christine Carter, Marilee Lin, Eleanor Brown, Jean Weiss, Phyllis Rogers, Katie Arnold, Christina Rivera Cogswell, Courtney Zenner Campbell, Joan Carol Lieberman, Brad Wetzler, Erin Wright, Sally Jordan, *Lighthouse* Writers

For mainstay strength: Katherine Halsey, Teresa Bowers Chapman, Heidi Zecher Burke, Sally Keefe, Kathryn Grody, Gideon Irving, Valentina Iturbe-LaGrave, Rodrigo Garcia, Reed Harwood, Aaron Slosberg, Simon Hart, Catherine Burgess, Andy Burgess, Lois Shannon, Tom Virden, Jen LeMaire, Will LeMaire, Joan Haug, Sven Haug, Jennifer Wright, Rebecca Bowie, Tania Schoennagel, Carrie O'Neill, Genny Horning, Laura Gunderson, Jane McClannan, Libby Foster, Todd Foster, Kristin Martindale

For light, wisdom, and helping hands: North street neighbors (best in the world), the Dragons' crew, the women of Avalanche Ranch, my students & colleagues from the Mountain School and the Thacher School, the MAIA team (change-makers), Midd '93, Gloo colleagues, readers of the *Brave over Perfect* blog (best-looking, wise, generous bunch), the TEDx Boulder team, Shana Kelly, Shannon O'Kane, Eva Vanek, Liz Wiig, Shannon Harriman, Sarah Byrden, Cate Brown, Marielle Reading, Salih Zain, Kim Hult, Jane Klein, Angela Merrill, Kylie Gettleman, Kyle Donahue, Shannon Lindow, Nancy Smith, Natalie Clements, Sarah Moorhouse, Anthony Moorhouse, Stewart McGrath, Debbie McGrath, Sarah Krakoff,

Karen Franklin, Mindy Caliguire, John Doyle, Ramon Schicchi, Susannah Clark, Andy Wasserman, Sarah Alexander, Liz Vautour, Jon Caliguire, Wende Valentine, Leo Eisenstein, Irene Li, Monique DeVane, Brian Driscoll, Alice and Chloe Zelkha

For nieces and nephews who show me how "b/p" is done: Aidan Caldwell, Celia Caldwell, Alex Rinehart, Katie Rinehart, Jon Rinehart, Blakley Dancy, Gabe Dancy, Zoë Caldwell, Jessie Caldwell, Hugo Caldwell

For everything: Kurt, Cole, and Hazel. Our family, and your love, give it all meaning and joy.

ABOUT THE AUTHOR

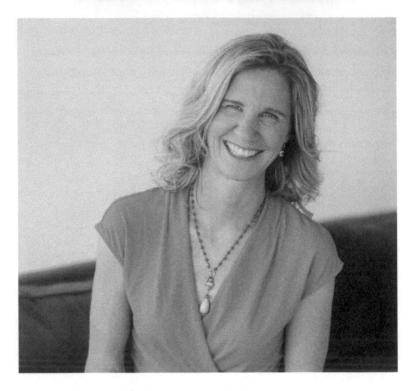

Susie Rinehart is a TEDx speaker, champion ultrarunner, mom, and brainstem tumor survivor. She began writing her blog from her hospital bed and is now an inspiration for those facing adversity. Her writing won her one of the highest prizes from the American Library Association. Susie now co-runs The Brave over Perfect Project, coaching leaders and organizations to proactively pursue risk and overcome perfectionism. Susie is also a champion of girls' education globally; a portion of the proceeds from the sale of *Fierce Joy* go to MAIA: Her Infinite Impact. She lives with her husband and children in Boulder, CO.